Coming Through
Depression

TONY BATES

Includes CD: A Mindful Approach to Recovery

Newleaf

Newleaf
an imprint of
Gill & Macmillan
Hume Avenue, Park West
Dublin 12
with associated companies throughout the world
www.gillmacmillan.ie

ISBN: 978 07171 4780 9

Index compiled by Róisín Nic Cóil
Design and print origination by O'K Graphic Design, Dublin
Printed and bound by CPI Group (UK) Ltd, Croydon, CR0 4YY

This book is typeset in 11/15 pt Minion
The paper used in this book comes from the wood pulp of managed forests.
For every tree felled, at least one tree is planted, thereby renewing natural
resources.

10 9 8

To my daughter Rachel, as you begin your career in clinical psychology.

May you find it as challenging and rewarding an adventure as I have.

Praise for Coming Through Depression

I am very grateful to Tony Bates for his deeply moving exploration of what depression means and feels for those who experience it and his clear steps to help people through it. It is a very empowering book, making it clear that depression need never have power over us because we ourselves and only we have the power in our own lives.

Tony writes in the language of the heart that bypasses the divide between academic and the street, a language that speaks directly to each of us.

The book is very personal but profoundly universal and in a positive way reminds us that the experience of depression can strengthen our sense of ourselves and help us become more aware and more appreciative of life.

The book is written with a radical simplicity without being simplistic and with deep sentiment without being sentimental. With great clarity it offers us the gift of mindfulness and the role it can play in the acceptance and recovery from depression.

SISTER STANISLAUS KENNEDY, VISIONARY AND SOCIAL INNOVATOR

This is a book full of gentle wisdom. Tony Bates invites the reader to begin, slowly and surely, to move through the darkest of times, through setbacks and false dawns, towards a genuine recovery. By bringing together ancient wisdom and modern scientific discoveries about what helps most, this book will be an invaluable guide to anyone who wishes to re-inhabit their life fully, with courage and self-compassion.

MARK WILLIAMS, DIRECTOR, UNIVERSITY OF OXFORD MINDFULNESS CENTRE

A powerful and erudite book, it is written in a clear style and will help many people; it's not just an essential manual for those struggling with depression, but also a road map for those seeking to find a path to a new and refreshed sense of selfhood.

MICHAEL HARDING, WRITER

Tony Bates, apart from being such a highly respected professional, has a wonderful rapport with our listeners. He has a particular empathy that communicates effortlessly on radio, perhaps because, as he says in this excellent book, 'I have battled through many a dark night of the soul myself'.

MARIAN FINUCANE, BROADCASTER

Acknowledgments

My thanks to my publisher, Michael Gill, for his invitation to rewrite and extend an earlier version of this book *Depression: A CommonSense Approach*. My understanding of depression has changed since I wrote this original work, and there are now new, effective ways to prevent depression recurring that had not been developed 10 years ago. In this book, I have incorporated many of the practical approaches to recovering from depression from the earlier work and I have extended them to introduce the reader to the practice of mindfulness, which offers unique possibilities for preventing recurrence of depression.

Particular thanks to Deirdre McHugh, for the sensitivity, creativity and rigour that she brought to editing this work. To those who gave me permission to include their stories in disguised form, and who cannot be named, my sincere thanks. My thanks also to Tim Symth for his critique of the final chapters on mindfulness and to my many teachers and friends who have shaped and clarified my understanding of depression and mindfulness, including Ursula Bates, Mark Williams, Jon Kabat-Zinn, Sr Stanislaus Kennedy, Michael Sanderson, David Whyte, John Welwood, Thich Nath Hahn, Paul Gilbert, Terry Lynch, Cathy Bache, Michael Ryan, Richard Hendrick, Aideen Loftus, Annafiona Keogh and Michael Lally, Aislinn Amory and Clive Shannon, thank you. My particular thanks to the young people with whom I work in Headstrong, who have taught me so much about the benefits of mindfulness training. Thank you also to my colleagues in Headstrong who helped with this book: Micheline Egan, Bob Illback, Blanaid Cleary, Helen Coughlan and Louize Carroll. Finally, thank you to Ola Mrozowska and her son, Michal.

The pain and brokenness of life that comes our way, does not in itself have the power to destroy us, because we have in us far greater power to heal and be made whole. It is strange but it is often only those who suffer greatly that are open to discovering the unbelievable power within. Another wonder of wonders is that those who find the inner power to let themselves be healed become more fully alive than those who have never experienced the depths of suffering.

Michael Ryan OCSO

Preface

I first wrote a version of this book 10 years ago, entitled *Depression: A CommonSense Approach.* In those 10 years, my understanding of depression has changed and matured. As I revisited the pages I had written, I encountered many places where my writing needed greater depth and clarity.

I am grateful to have had the chance to revisit this project and particularly to include a brand-new section on mindfulness. Mindfulness has been shown to offer a powerful protection to people who are vulnerable to depression. I believe this book offers the reader a much fuller account of the path to recovery.

Our lives are interwoven with emotions of all kinds, every day. There are no negative emotions or positive emotions. All emotions offer pathways to understanding ourselves more and more each day, and this understanding enables us to make sense of the world in which we live.

When the way we feel becomes hard for us to accept, when we are having repetitive thoughts about how negative we are as a person, and when we cannot seem to shift this thinking and we feel worn down and at a loss as to how to live in the world, we describe this experience as depression.

Depression is a word we use very loosely, as though it were exactly the same experience for everyone. In fact, it is very particular to each person who feels that way. No single person will feel exactly the same way as another who feels overwhelmed and unhappy in themselves.

Mindfulness means paying attention to whatever is happening in the present moment, and accepting our experience without judging it or trying to fix or change anything. It invites us to relate to our experience with kindness instead of reacting to it and getting carried away by stories about how we 'shouldn't be' feeling this way. Practising mindfulness helps us to calm down, to become more aware of what is going on within us, and to meet our difficulties with honesty and acceptance.

What if the way you feel right now is the only way you can feel in this particular moment? What if this moment doesn't get any better than it is right now? What if it were possible to hold our experience in awareness and allow it to be just the way it already is?

That would be an incredibly radical act, says Jon Kabat-Zinn, a pioneer in mindfulness training, but it would also be an act of profound wisdom. We would stop struggling against the way things are. We would start to investigate what is happening and see that inside of our sadness, our grief and our despair, there is something else going on; some kind of deep understanding in us that recognises that loss is real for all of us, that disappointment is inevitable, that everything is changing, that our bodies age, and that we can't control the universe, much as we would like to.

And this is not all black, because we have evolved over billions of years to deal precisely with this type of reality. There is no other reality. We are fragile and we can be broken – but we also have within us a capacity to adapt, to be changed and to evolve through facing our difficulties.

For many of us, it is hard to stop and take time to step into the present moment. Our mind is always on the way to somewhere else. We blast through our days and weeks, living somewhere in the future a lot of the time . We tell ourselves that we will only be able to settle in the present when the conditions are right, but of course they are never right.

The truth is that we don't believe that we can find happiness in the present moment. In fact, we are more likely to believe that we will only find happiness if we steer clear of the present.

Maybe we are afraid of what we might find there – unpleasant and painful feelings that we fear could overwhelm us – and we would rather push them out of our minds and steer clear of them. We may even be reluctant to stop and appreciate pleasant experiences, because we always imagine there will be an even better time, somewhere in the future, when everything will be just the way we want it, and when we can be *really* happy.

So we tend to live lives where we constantly distract ourselves. We worry or fantasise about what might happen, or we brood over the past, regretting what has happened, running it over and over in our minds as if somehow by doing this we can change the past. Living this way can be exhausting.

Some part of us would like to stop running, to come home to the present moment and rest there, but we don't know how.

The practice of mindfulness helps us to find a place of quiet in our lives, where we can feel safe and steady ourselves. When we learn to rest in the present moment, we are able to be with whatever we are feeling without being overwhelmed and without getting carried away by our fearful thoughts.

This revised version of my earlier book, *Depression: A CommonSense Approach*, takes you on a journey that involves looking courageously at what happens when you feel depressed and are listening to what it may be trying to tell you about your life. This forms Part One of this book. Part Two gives you some guidance as to how you can get back on your feet and regain some control over your life, so that you don't continue to feel lost. Putting some structure on your everyday life is necessary so that you can relate to your deeper hurts and wounds. Part Three introduces you to the practice of mindfulness and shows you how you can live with yourself and begin to heal those places in your mind and heart where you remain vulnerable to depression. You will be introduced to specific ways that will help you to rest in the present, pay attention to what is happening in your body and find stability. When you have taken time to practise these skills, you will be able to be open to painful emotions and thoughts without becoming overwhelmed. These exercises can prevent you from slipping back into an experience of depression, which can be a very demoralising and heart-breaking experience for anyone who feels they have already put depression behind them.

It is possible for any human being to 'lose their way', but it is equally possible for any human being to 'find their way'. When we feel lost, it is not because of what's happening or what is missing in our life; we only feel lost when we cannot see what is happening and when we become too frightened to be with ourselves. The moment you can name what is there and be with your experience, you will not feel so lost.

Being mindful, being present to ourselves, connects us with our inner strength. We discover that no matter how broken we may feel, we are also fully human and whole, and we have an amazing capacity to hold and transform whatever is happening in our awareness, with compassion.

Recovery is a path that each of us follows as we engage more openly and more courageously with the life we have been given. Your path to recovery is not something that anyone can point out to you. It is something you discover, one step at a time, and it always begins with the place you are in right now. Mindfulness can help us to see beyond the noise level of our thoughts to the supports that are available to us, and clear a space in our mind where new insights can emerge.

The way ahead is particular to each person as they learn what works for them and what enables them to be themselves. Some parts of this book may be especially meaningful to one reader and not so relevant to another. I have divided it into three distinct parts that stand alone and which can be read in any order, depending on the particular difficulty a person may be facing.

Depression is not a power in our lives. We ourselves are the power in our lives. When we forget that and when we believe we are worthless, we lose sight of where we are going. By rediscovering the power in ourselves, we rediscover the will to live life in a more meaningful way, and we learn to love ourselves again in a deeper way.

I hope that you will find in these pages an understanding of depression that not only helps you to overcome the pain of depression, but that also helps you to learn how to live your life. May it help you to become more aware of places in your heart that need to heal, give you the confidence to face whatever frightens you, and enable you to discover the freedom to be yourself more fully.

Tony Bates
May 2011

Contents

Introduction

Susan was tall, blonde and in her late twenties. Her outward appearance suggested a self-contained, confident woman, but her eyes told a different story. The day she first arrived, she looked as if she'd rather have been anywhere else than talking to me. Her movements were awkward and stiff. She avoided making eye contact and I hesitated to ask her why she'd come, sensing it might be an invasion of a privacy that she was anxiously guarding. We danced around the central issue for a while as I pieced together a profile of her family background, her schooling and occupation, and her current circumstances. She relaxed a little but when I asked what had brought her to see me, her fragile holding together gave way to a flood of tears.

Words failed Susan as she tried vainly to account for her terrible sadness. She felt she had no right to complain but she described how in recent weeks she had found herself collapsing into tears for no apparent reason, overcome by the feeling that she was stupid, worthless and completely out of control. She apologised repeatedly for her demeanour.

She struck me as someone who didn't normally, if ever, let down her guard about her inner struggles. But on this occasion the intensity of her inner pain refused to be silenced and she had sought counselling to help her make some sense of it all.

In writing this book, I think about Susan on that first visit, and many others who have come and confronted their own very personal experience of depression. All have been confused and frightened by what was happening to them. Their own desperation, the experience of 'losing a grip' on work and life, or the helpless exasperation of close loved ones, prompted them to reach out and look for help.

I imagine you are reading this book having struggled also with depression, either directly or indirectly, through living with someone who is visited and revisited by this problem. My hope is that you will find in Susan's story, and in the accounts of others' struggles with depression, some echo of your own experience, and realise that you are not 'mad' or 'stupid' or 'horribly selfish'.

There are reasons why someone becomes depressed; being able to understand and make sense of the experience can help to restore one's dignity and morale. There are also ways to recover from depression and stay well that this book will describe in some detail. And there are ways in which the experience of depression can strengthen your sense of who you are and help you become more aware and appreciative of your life.

Depression is challenging for families and loved ones. Children may sense and feel troubled by a parent's dark moods; partners even more so. The effort to alleviate the pain of depression in a loved one inevitably fails, and the most well-intended interventions of friends and spouses can leave all concerned feeling helpless and alienated. While this book is primarily intended as a guide to recovery for the sufferer, it is also written with the relatives and friends of the sufferer in mind, in the hope that it may make sense of what can be a difficult problem to grasp from the 'outside'. An understanding of the problem, by all who are affected, can act as a bridge between people who feel isolated by depression and those who care about them.

The aim of this book is to support and strengthen your recovery from depression. Recovery is not just about feeling better. It means getting to know yourself in a much deeper way than you do now and learning how best to take care of yourself. Your faith in yourself may be shaky right now, but my hope is that in this book you will find a way to connect with your own inner strength.

You might well ask whether I am being realistic in thinking that a simple book like this could change your life in such a profound way. Let me say this first so neither of us has any illusions: nobody can magically take away another's depression. I can only join with someone who is in this particular pain and help them to discover in themselves a capacity to heal and to confront their pain rather than try to block it out or become overwhelmed by it.

If you are struggling with depression right now, you need a solid ally to help you find your way back home. And, as allies go, it turns out I'm not the worst. I've worked with many people for over 25 years to help them recover from depression and I have battled through many a dark night of the soul myself. Like a tracker who knows the territory, I can help to guide you and direct you to useful strategies that may help your recovery.

At the same time, I recognise that a book like this one is no substitute to you finding a trustworthy professional to work with during your recovery. Self-help literature is often most useful when it is used as part of a recovery plan that may well include medication and/or therapy. We will talk more about this later, but do consider engaging someone competent to help you find your way out of depression. Your GP can advise you on how best to start looking for the right person. One of the benefits of reading this book is that it may help to clarify what kind of help you need.

Sarah, whose journals we will be dipping in and out of throughout this book, was a young woman with whom I worked. When we first met, she was 21 years old and in a very dark place. With her permission, I have included excerpts from the journal she kept over the course of five months, when, as an in-patient, she struggled to find a way out of depression. I learned a great deal from Sarah, and from many others whose accounts of recovery I have also included in these pages.

Sarah's recovery journal

Excerpt 1

Depression is like an assignment in life that nobody ever sets for you to do. No one tells you beforehand how difficult it's going to be, how time-consuming it is, how painful it can be. You're not prepared for it and when it happens, you want to give it all away and collapse into nothing. Because there are no real signs, no real markers, no sheets handed out beforehand, telling you what it's going to be like. And before you know it, you're being judged, not on your progress but on your failures, on your weaknesses. The judge isn't a fair one with guidelines and suggestions. The judge is yourself, the 'worst' around, who shatters your confidence and who plays on your vulnerabilities until you get to the point where you want to break. You want to give up on this assignment that seems so wasteful and pointless.

But it's really the most important assignment you'll be given. It's an essay which is long and tiresome but where you must come out with full marks. Those full marks won't be given for content or structure or quality. They'll be given each time you believe in yourself and care for yourself a little more. And you're the one who calls out the grade, because you're the one giving yourself those stars. The assignment is you, and you are the judge, the expert, the one who knows you and cares about you and loves you enough to say, 'I'm worth it, I'm worth 100 per cent.'

PART ONE

Understanding Depression

CHAPTER 1

The experience of depression

*Depression! Depression is not a word that for a long time I
would have applied to myself. In retrospect, however, I would
probably now accept that I have been depressed over a long
number of years and in need of some help.*

Mary, aged 39

Depression is a very common term that many people can
relate to in some way. We have all had our share of losses
and felt sad; we have all made mistakes and experienced
disappointments and setbacks. These experiences may have left
us feeling upset and confused. They may have been quite
shattering and taken some time to get over. So we know what it's
like to feel sadness and distress and we may wonder what makes
our experience any different from what is referred to as
'depression' in a clinical or medical sense.

When someone feels sad, or when they experience a passing,
depressed mood, it is generally a normal and healthy response to
some misfortune they have experienced. Most of the time, their
mood is a reaction to the loss of a person, a social role, a close
companion or a place to which they felt attached. A person who
feels sad knows they have lost something and they yearn for its
return. Generally, they will share their grief with someone and
be open to receiving whatever support they get as they come to
terms with their loss. For a period of time, they will grieve until
they can gradually accept their loss. Their emotional life and their

capacity to work and relate to others may be temporarily disrupted. This is a natural part of coming to terms with the new situation they find themselves in and learning to re-engage with life without whomever or whatever they have lost.

Depression is something different. Whereas sadness and grief are focused entirely around an experience of loss, depression refers to an experience where a person becomes convinced that there is something seriously wrong with them. If sadness is a natural response to loss, depression is a very painful experience of believing oneself to be a 'loser'. In depression, a person's distress may have been triggered by some loss in their life, but their attention very quickly shifts away from whatever they have lost to a preoccupation with a personal sense of failure, inadequacy and helplessness. Lacking any belief that they are worthwhile, they may turn away from others and become withdrawn and unresponsive to offers of help.

When someone becomes depressed, it is not simply that they feel down. Their capacity to think clearly and make decisions is diminished, their physical health suffers, and the energy they normally have to deal with life drains away. A person who becomes depressed also experiences a complete lack of satisfaction from the activities, relationships and pastimes that had always given their lives a sense of meaning and joy.

Because depression can be so disabling and so intensely painful, it is regarded as being as much of an illness as any other form of physical suffering. It can last for a long time and a person may feel utterly hopeless about whether or not they will ever recover. When depression persists for a long time, a person may begin to feel that they are an intolerable burden to others and convince themselves that everyone might be better off if they were no longer around.

This book is about the experience of feeling down that seems to take hold of us, that doesn't shift easily and that causes us significant difficulty in getting through our everyday lives.

This experience is commonly referred to as clinical depression and it is as much a physical experience as it is an emotional experience. Clinical depression causes us such difficulty that it becomes extremely hard for us to live our lives in a way that we want for ourselves. People who become clinically depressed may feel confused, terrified and fearful and no longer in charge of their own lives.

In the early stage of her depression, Sarah described her experience in her journal. Her account conveys the sense of confusion and isolation so characteristic of depression.

Sarah's recovery journal

Excerpt 2

These days, I don't know what to do with my time. Almost everything seems so futile, nothing seems to have any importance any more. I don't feel really depressed all the time, just bogged down with living. I spend a lot of time in a daze, as though I'm hiding things from myself; my memory is blocked, my feelings are blocked and I feel like a walking stone statue. Some of the time, I think I feel OK, but then my mood changes and I become frightened again. I move back on occasions during the day to those so familiar periods of despair when inside my head I can hear myself screaming, 'Help me, what am I supposed to do?'

Signs of depression

Depression is characterised by a particular set of changes in how a person thinks, feels and behaves. As well as being an experience of intense psychological suffering, a person's sense of physical wellbeing is greatly affected, and sleep, appetite and energy levels are all disturbed. The primary signs or 'symptoms' of depression are discussed below and illustrated in the diagram below. The symptoms in this diagram are categorised and grouped according to their impact on our thinking and our feeling, and on our behaviours and our physical health.

SYMPTOMS OF DEPRESSION

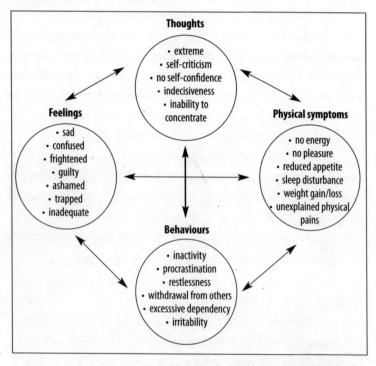

Ways of thinking that are characteristic of depression

As Tim describes below, a person who is depressed thinks about their world in a very negative way.

You're in a café, you're talking to someone and you're not even able to listen to what they're saying: the other customers' cups grate too loudly on their saucers, you're worried you've offended the waitress because you forgot to say 'please', and of course you don't want your mate to realise you're not paying attention. Everything ends up stewed down to its component fibres because you're looking at it all so hard. You're seeing too much and too deeply, and holding all those details together in your mind is taking up all of your effort.

John, aged 21

The past, the present and the future are all viewed though a dark lens that distorts everything. Important achievements in the past don't count. She or he focuses exclusively on every sign of failure or weakness that they can possibly point to in their life. They see the future as a relentless continuation of their current misery where nothing good will ever happen for them. These preoccupations make it hard to concentrate on anything or to believe there is any good in themselves. Making a decision can be an enormous strain because they don't trust themselves to do the right thing.

Sarah, in her darkest moments of depression, described how her sense of hopelessness was overwhelming.

Sarah's recovery journal

Excerpt 3

I can't do anything any more. Anytime I attempt to work, I clog up inside and leave it. I don't do anything because I don't think that I can. There's no point, it's all so hopeless. Even if I do try, I get nowhere. I have absolutely no belief in myself any more. There's no hope in my heart, there's no happiness in my thoughts. I feel as if I'm tied up and can't break loose. I'm too afraid to do anything because I think I'll fail and it'll only make me feel worse, and so I do nothing. But that makes me feel so bad because all I do is sit around and do nothing. I'm so lazy. I don't understand anything. What's the point?

> It's all so useless, and worthless and utterly hopeless and I hate it. I'm so afraid.

Other people very often view people who are depressed as being terribly 'selfish'. While it is true that their thoughts seem to centre exclusively on themselves, and that their behaviour might seem very self-centred, it is not accurate to say they are 'selfish'. Such pain is generated within the mind when a person is depressed that the person is often unable to consider the needs of others or to contribute to activities where they would normally play an active role.

The physical symptoms of depression

Depression is for many people a very physical experience and the symptoms they describe are often to do with changes in their body. They may describe the sensation of hurting deeply inside or they may have physical symptoms which worry them, but which have no apparent physical cause. Sleep disturbance is probably the most common physical symptom of depression. Sufferers usually report a broken sleep pattern that results in waking without the sense of being rested or refreshed. Their normal appetite may also be affected, resulting in either excessive eating and weight gain, or a complete lack of interest in food, which leads to weight loss. They may also find themselves unable to make love and indeed have very little interest in doing so, and this can be a major worry for them.

Behavioural characteristics of depression

It is not always easy to recognise that someone may be depressed. No matter how intensely distressed they may feel inside, many people hide it very well on the outside. And even when someone behaves out of character, we may not realise that they are depressed, and mistake their behaviour for something else.

This is often the case with children and adolescents who may express their inner turmoil in behaviour that appears destructive and anti-social. For example, an adolescent may begin to act in an uncharacteristic way, participating in shoplifting, fire-setting or disruptive behaviour at school, and never get the support for what is really troubling them. An adult's sudden lack of interest in sexual intimacy may be interpreted as rejection, or they may start to drink heavily and procrastinate and get into trouble for not delivering on their work responsibilities. All of these behaviours result in life being more difficult for anyone experiencing depression and can reinforce their belief that they are fundamentally bad.

A significant slowing down in activity is a very common feature of depression, although some sufferers can become restless, even hyperactive, as they try to block out the turmoil they experience inside. Excessive 'busy-ness' can be a protective mechanism to distract from this turmoil, but it leaves a person feeling constantly on edge and irritable. Sometimes being busy can seem preferable to the prospect of slowing down and acknowledging that something is not right. Susan, who was mentioned in the introduction, put this very succinctly when she said, 'You make yourself very vulnerable when you stop to think!'

Most commonly, the behaviour that is characteristic of depression is marked by lack of energy and social withdrawal. One man in his mid-thirties, described how his 'get-up-and-go was all gone'. There is little energy to devote to external demands and concerns when you are depressed. A tendency to take to the bed is all too common. Sometimes it can seem easier just to retreat from the world to avoid having to deal with the criticism, demands, even concerns, of loved ones and friends.

Feelings that are characteristic of depression

If you have never been depressed, it is hard to appreciate just how intensely painful depression can feel. People who are depressed often find it very hard to put their feelings into words. They also fear that if they were to say how badly they were feeling, other people may be shocked and write them off as insane. Sarah described the feeling of being depressed in the following way:

> I'm so distressed because I don't know what's going on in my head. It's confusing and I feel frightened and unsure about everything I do. I used to be happy and cheerful and confident. I used to enjoy my life. Where has everything gone? I don't understand why I feel like this, why I feel so worn out, sad and lonely. I need warmth. I need to be warmed up inside. Everything's gone cold and strange. I'd love for someone to give me a big hug, but if I asked, I feel that they wouldn't understand why and that they would think I was crazy.

Emotions can be so intense when you're depressed that you can become frightened of your inner world. You do whatever you can to suppress your feelings and block them out. Your body may become tense with the worry about what you are feeling. Or you may resort to abusing alcohol or other substances to shut down your feelings and make yourself as numb as possible.

Severe and mild depression

Depression may be experienced to a mild, moderate or severe degree. In its mild or moderate forms, it is characterised by negative thinking and low self-esteem, irritability, and difficulty in concentrating. If this state of mind continues over an extended period of time (at least one year), the individual is deemed to be suffering from what is termed 'dysthymia', which is a low-grade form of depression that endures for a long period and can easily go unnoticed.

In the more severe forms of depression, the same symptoms are experienced with greater intensity and physical manifestations of this distress are more apparent. Symptoms of fatigue, insomnia or hypersomnia (too little or too much sleep), decreased or increased appetite, significant change in weight, and a marked slowing down of physical and mental activity, indicate the need for professional help. Suicidal thoughts often lurk just beneath the surface and should always be checked for and regarded with the utmost seriousness. A diagnosis of severe, or major, depression is applicable if the majority of these symptoms are experienced every day for at least *two weeks.*

Bipolar or manic depression refers to severe episodes of depression that are interspersed with at least one episode of elation or mania. A pattern of mood swings is observable over time, where the above symptoms of major depression can alternate with the individual experiencing extreme agitation where their thinking may be speeded up and their mood elated. During these 'high' episodes, the sufferer may exhibit pressured speech, inappropriate behaviour that is out of character for them, and beliefs that are compelling for the sufferer, but unreasonable to everyone else.

Recognising depression in children and adolescents

The most frequent ages for people to experience depression for the first time is between 13–15 years old. This is a disturbing statistic because it suggests that young people experience depression at a time in life when they are least able to cope with it. Medication may help in extreme situations but a lot more support is required if we are to teach these teenagers the skills to live their lives and build their self-confidence to face the issues that may be causing their depression.

There has been increasing attention in recent years on the growing incidence of depression in childhood and adolescence. One study of 3,000 schoolchildren found that 5 per cent of the group was reporting mild to moderate depression. Chronic marital conflict, neglect, parental rejection or serious stresses in adjusting to school often account for such reactions in children. Sadness, anxiety and fearfulness may characterise childhood depression, but the experience of these young people is often reflected in poor schoolwork and aggressive behaviour which may mislead adults into thinking that these children are simply misbehaving.

The same criteria used above to diagnose depression in adults have been found to apply to children and young people, but with certain modifications. For example, studies find that four out of five children who are depressed are more likely to come across as irritable rather than sad. Children also tend to externalise their suffering in the form of disruptive behaviour, which can result in them being perceived as having 'behaviour problems'. This behaviour can be an expression of their anger at life for having let them down in some way. Whereas adults are more inclined to blame themselves for feeling depressed, a young person is more likely to believe that 'life sucks' and to take it out on others in whatever way they can. They may have their own good reasons for feeling this way, but the problem is that their anti-social behaviour may be the only thing people see when they come to the attention of adults, and the underlying feelings of hurt and confusion that fuels their behaviour may be completely overlooked. As a result, these children may be punished rather than supported.

Some researchers have found that children who are depressed, especially pre-schoolers and pre-adolescents, are unlikely to report feeling sad and hopeless but instead can tend to 'look' depressed in both their facial expression and their posture. When children reach the age of adolescence, their depressed mood becomes similar to that of adults. They will report feeling depressed and often complain of physical symptoms that bother them. With older teenagers, depression is often likely to co-exist with eating disorders and substance abuse disorders. Other symptoms that are noted are social withdrawal, excessive worrying and conduct problems.

Suicidal thoughts and self-harm attempts are very common in about two-thirds of young people who feel depressed. Studies have reported actual suicide attempts in 6–12 per cent of depressed children and young adolescents. These rates appear to be higher among young people than among depressed adults. In Ireland, the high incidence of suicide and self-harm in the 15–24-year age group has become a source of alarm. It signals that while many of our young people may be doing well in their lives, there is a significant percentage of young people who may be in crisis and need our support.

Depression during pregnancy or following childbirth

The experience of pregnancy and raising a baby is a basic and fundamental part of human life. It is something that takes place every day and is considered to be one of the most natural events that a woman can experience. However, this can lead to an assumption that every woman is emotionally prepared for all the changes that pregnancy and childbirth bring to her life. The truth is that while many women cope well with the physical challenges of pregnancy and childbirth, many others can find the experience stressful and emotionally challenging.

The period during pregnancy and after childbirth is for many women a time of increased vulnerability to depression.

Depression is experienced by 8–15% of women within one year of childbirth and is often referred to as 'postnatal depression'. This experience is more often accompanied by feelings of anxiety and it can feel relentless and exhausting. A woman may be unable to see a future where she does not feel this way. She may doubt whether she will ever be able to have another child.

A new mother may feel very ashamed of feeling this way. She may have always believed that childbirth was a 'natural' experience, one that she imagined every other woman welcomes. She may compare herself to friends or sisters who had babies and who delighted in them. She is reluctant to admit that for her, her feelings for this child are more confused. She may be reluctant to say how she feels to anyone, fearful perhaps that others may regard her as ungrateful or incapable of raising this child. While the new baby captivates everyone's attention, no one sees her suffering and this can make her feel alone and trapped.

The term 'postnatal depression' was coined to describe this experience, because it appeared that in most cases a woman suddenly experienced depression following childbirth. However, recent research has shown that 'postnatal depression' is very often the continuation of an experience that began during pregnancy. Perhaps because a woman assumed that her low mood was part of the normal experience of pregnancy and didn't think to seek support for how she was feeling, her distress was not picked up on until after she had given birth.

Since the antenatal and postnatal period up to a year after birth are referred to as the 'perinatal' period, the terms 'perinatal mental health' and 'perinatal depression' have now become more common among researchers and clinicians.

Why might the arrival of a child make someone feel depressed?

What gives rise to this painful experience of depression in some women? When you consider the number of challenges that come with having a child and how vulnerable a woman may feel as she prepares to bring a new child into the world, the fact that one in ten women experience depression should not come as a complete surprise.

For example, the arrival of a child can bring new challenges in her relationship with her partner. A woman is immediately required to provide constant care for her baby and she may have to make changes in her work role to allow her to care for the baby.

The belief that being a mother is 'instinctive', 'easy' and 'joyful' may make it all the harder for a woman to admit to herself or anyone else that she is finding the whole experience overwhelming. She may assume that if she does not feel happy, it must be because she lacks something, or that she doesn't have what it takes to be a 'good' mother.

How well a partner adjusts to the arrival of a child can also have a profound effect on how the mother might feel. At a time when a woman may be isolated due to the work involved in caring for a child, she may become more dependent than usual on her family and her partner for support. Women with supportive partners who give them empathy and encouragement feel better about themselves. But for women with relationships where there is frequent conflict or very little communication, they can feel very isolated and cut off from the practical and emotional support they need.

Any loss of energy or difficulty in concentrating makes all of these tasks all the more challenging.

RISK FACTORS FOR DEVELOPING PERINATAL DEPRESSION

Despite a large amount of research, no single causative factor has been identified to account for the distress that some women experience. A number of specific 'risk' factors have been identified that place a woman at risk for depression. These include:

- A tendency to punish oneself for not measuring up to expectations
- Expectations that women have of themselves regarding how they 'should' feel about the birth of a child
- Lack of a partner and social support
- A traumatic birth
- Episodes of depression or anxiety during the pregnancy
- Patterns of thinking, including a habit of dwelling on negative events.

What helps women who feel depressed during pregnancy or following childbirth?

In 1960, the first study to explore the benefit of mental health education with women who were pregnant was carried out and revealed something interesting about what might be happening to women during this time in their lives. A group of women were randomly assigned to one of two classes during their pregnancy, one that provided some guidelines on looking after their mental health and the other some more general information about pregnancy. The women who attended the mental health class experienced significantly less 'emotional upset' after they had given birth compared with the others. Furthermore, those who were accompanied by their partners had the best outcome.

Despite this pioneering study, there was little research into what could help to prevent mental health difficulties until the turn of the millennium. Research concentrated instead on searching for the hormonal causes and treatments of postnatal depression. While intuitively we may believe that hormones must be involved in perinatal depression, the fact is that forty years of research has failed to prove that hormones 'cause' this experience. What has been shown to be the case, however, is that social and personal difficulties in a woman's life (see table titled 'Risk factors for developing perinatal depression') can give rise to depression.

The danger in seeing this experience as completely hormonal is that we may fail to address the real difficulties in a woman's life that have given rise to her depression. Medication may have a limited role in the management of perinatal depression, but what matters most to a woman is that someone is willing to take the time to understand what the experience of giving birth has been for her, to understand what would make her feel better about herself and what supports she needs to raise her child.

Checking your mood

What have you learned from the above? Do you recognise something of your own experience of depression? Perhaps you have been afraid to acknowledge that something is wrong. Hopefully what you've read so far has made it easier for you to understand what is going on in your life. This is not to say your problems have been solved, but that you can name what is happening, no matter how painful that may be. It may be that the place you're in is extremely difficult, and that you are experiencing depression, that you've realised how real your problems actually are, and that you are now in a position to begin to address those problems. It is also possible that you are not depressed, but that you are hurting in your life because of the challenges you are trying to face that are difficult and painful.

Sometimes we need to stop and be honest with ourselves about the reality of our lives, in order to identify the strains that are affecting us, and to start taking some new steps to deal with them. Often, doing something, which may be very small or simple, can make a big difference towards easing the pain of our difficulties.

The list below identifies the 12 most common symptoms of depression. To help you clarify what your experience of depression may or may not be, look at each symptom and tick 'Yes' to any of the symptoms that describe how you have been feeling, for most of the time, over the past two weeks (or longer).

CHECKLIST OF THE MOST COMMON SYMPTOMS OF DEPRESSION

Indicate which of the following, if any, you've experienced over the past two weeks by ticking yes or no.	YES	NO
1. I have been feeling down most of the time.	___	___
2. I get no pleasure from the things that normally mean a lot to me.	___	___
3. I feel tired all the time.	___	___
4. I can't concentrate and remember details.	___	___
5. I have lost weight quite dramatically.	___	___
6. My sleep is disturbed and doesn't leave me feeling rested.	___	___
7. I am more irritable than usual.	___	___
8. I have lost all confidence in my ability to make decisions.	___	___
9. My thoughts are mostly self-critical and gloomy.	___	___
10. I feel guilty without really knowing why.	___	___
11. I feel sensations in my body that trouble me.	___	___
12. I have thoughts of killing myself.	___	___

If you have ticked 'Yes' to either of the first two items and 'Yes' to at least four of the remaining items, this suggests that you may be experiencing depression. The higher the number of items you ticked, the more severe your depression.

Pay particular attention to your answer to question 12, the last item on the checklist, which relates to suicidal thoughts. While it is common for people who are depressed to think that everything would be somehow easier if they were dead, it is important to emphasise that if these thoughts are more than just occasional, or if they have progressed to where you are actively thinking about ways to 'end it all', then it is imperative that you seek some professional help, or contact one of the helplines at the end of this book. Your GP is probably the most appropriate and accessible person for you to consult because he or she can direct you to someone who can help.

Who gets depressed?

It is estimated that about 20 per cent of us become clinically depressed at some point in our lives. This figure seems to have stayed the same over the past 50 years. When you consider that people are experiencing depression earlier and earlier in their lives, and that it recurs in over half of those who experience it, then it is clear that there are far more people suffering from depression on any given day, than one might realise.

One remarkably consistent finding in studies across different continents has been that women are about twice as likely to experience depression as men. The highest incidence of depression in women is among those in the 20–40-year age group. However, men and women become depressed in equal numbers where they are in similar roles, such as in student life or in professional careers.

In spite of its frequency, only one in 10 of the people who become depressed seek professional help. Sometimes this is simply because people do not know where to turn for help, but, for many, their lack of help-seeking is because they feel ashamed, and they fear how others will judge them if it comes out that they had any kind of 'mental health' problem. The stigma that has surrounded talking about mental health is lifting as we speak more openly about the way mental suffering touches all our lives and hear from people who have recovered from all kinds of mental health difficulties. We are beginning to see how experiences like depression can deepen our lives and make us more compassionate towards ourselves and others.

Summary
Depression has some universal characteristics but each person experiences slightly different combinations of symptoms. For some, it is an intensely physical experience and affects their energy level and overall sense of wellbeing. Others can somehow keep going but their hyperactivity is often an attempt to run away from their inner lives. Some sufferers are prone to long spells of inner torment as they are overwhelmed by negative thoughts and feelings of tremendous personal failure. If this distress continues over a long period, their ability to function is inevitably compromised. Personal relationships can become severely strained, and work colleagues may notice them being edgy, falling behind, procrastinating on important projects or withdrawing from the company of others. However it is sparked, depression is confusing and frightening for the sufferer and life can be an extremely isolating and lonely experience at that time.

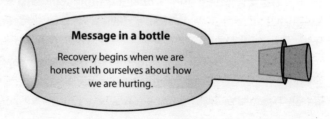

Message in a bottle

Recovery begins when we are honest with ourselves about how we are hurting.

CHAPTER 2

What causes depression?

Many people experience difficulties in their childhood that trouble them in their adult lives. The experiences of loss, separation, neglect or abuse can result in trauma that we feel in our bodies. We may try to push the memory of these experiences away into the deepest recesses of our minds and continue to live and manage our daily lives. One day, however, something happens that stirs up feelings associated with these memories and we start to feel uneasy in ourselves and to doubt that we can control the feelings that have been stirred up. When painful experiences in life trigger deep insecurities and fears inside ourselves, we become vulnerable to depression.

When our deepest insecurities and self-doubts are stirred, we are often surprised by the intensity of our reactions and wonder why we are feeling the way we do. The trigger can be something that another person might brush off as insignificant, but it awakens in us a deep pain that we have been suppressing for many years.

We may feel very lost and unsure of how to proceed in our lives when this happens. We worry that we are 'losing it' or 'going mad' or having some kind of 'breakdown'. We find it hard to cope with day-to-day demands and it becomes hard just to make it through the day. Our most natural reaction is to try to shut out the distress we are feeling inside, to ignore the confusion in our minds and to do whatever it takes to shut out the pain. These strategies may buy us some time but eventually our pain catches up with us.

Depression begins to spread across our inner world when we decide that there must be something wrong with us for feeling the way we do. We blame ourselves for the grief and sorrow that has been awakened inside us. We go around and around inside our minds, convincing ourselves that we are 'weak', 'pathetic' and 'useless' and that there is nothing we can ever do to change the way we are.

Recovery begins when we recognise the pain we are in. We may not understand why we are reacting so sensitively to whatever triggered the crisis we find ourselves in, but with time and some help, we can figure it out. Meanwhile we can give ourselves the benefit of the doubt and be kind to ourselves rather than critical. By accepting that our inner lives are complex and that we are not to blame for the way we feel, we take one more step on the path to recovery.

Let's look at what a century of psychological research has identified as some of the reasons why we become depressed.

Early childhood experiences that leave us vulnerable to depression

When we are children, we are immensely fragile and utterly dependent on the care and protection of others. When we are loved and offered warmth in a consistent way, we feel secure and our whole body expresses gratitude and affection. But our dependence on others also leaves us vulnerable. If our parents or carers are not able to be there for us, or if they are there one moment and not there the next, we feel anxious. As a child, we do not understand that the behaviour of our parents or carers reflects their personal limitations. We imagine their behaviour must have something to do with who we are, or that there is something that we are doing that makes them behave in the way they do. By the time the mind has been able to comprehend what may have happened, the wounds of the heart are already too deep.

A consistently conflicted relationship between a child and their parents can set the stage for depression. Very often the harshness that permeates a parent's way of relating to their children directly reflects the lack of affection that they themselves received as children. As a result of their own difficult upbringing, parents or carers may not feel able to respond comfortably to their own children's emotional needs, and so they may discourage affection-seeking or dependent behaviour. Children can experience this distancing as rejection, and they can carry the memory of those feelings in their bodies right into their adult lives. These memories of rejection can undermine their confidence to engage in meaningful relationships with others. They do not find intimacy easy and they fear that if someone discovered who they really were, they would surely be rejected.

These feelings of insecurity and self-doubt can prevent them from opening up to other people in their adult lives, and they may feel unable to ask others for help, at times in their life when they are most in need of support.

When young people who are depressed are asked about their relationships with their parents, they generally describe themselves as not feeling close or able to talk to them openly about how they are feeling. They often describe their mothers and fathers as rejecting, controlling and as showing very little warmth. Looking more closely at relationships within families that appeared to set children up for becoming depressed, studies have repeatedly identified two characteristics: 'low affection' and 'high control'. Parents who show little warmth and who set high standards, and parents who are harshly critical in an attempt to get their children to meet their high expectations, produce children who tend to berate themselves and think of themselves as failures.

Some people believe that children are not affected by these experiences, that they 'get used' to them and brush them off. Nothing could be further from the truth. While children may well develop a protective front and act as though they couldn't care less about their parents' behaviour, sooner or later their true feelings of hurt and pain emerge, either in the form of anger towards others or hatred towards themselves. They often expect to be rejected and, as adults, they may find any encounter with someone who accepts them hard to take. They may test that person's acceptance by doing everything they can to provoke their rejection.

The most striking characteristic of people who are prone to depression is their belief that there is something fundamentally bad or unlovable about them as human beings. The phrase 'having a poor self-image' is often used to describe this state of mind, but it does little to capture how intensely painful it can be to feel this way. 'Self-loathing' probably comes closer to expressing how someone who feels depressed thinks about themselves.

Trauma and separation in our early life can also affect our sense of feeling safe in the world. The loss of a parent, severe illness and hospitalisation all leave their mark on a child. Numerous studies have found that depression can be related to the loss of a parent in early childhood. When something happens in our adult life that feels in any way similar to our early experience, we can find ourselves suddenly reliving the way we felt as young children.

This finding is not meant to imply that loss and separation in childhood always has a long-term negative impact. What matters is how the child was cared for following a loss and not simply that the loss happened. The experience of depression can be associated with experiences of loss that were followed by lack of any consistent care or attention for the child, or the lack of an effort to help them to make sense of their confusion.

Rigid rules of living

Children are amazingly resilient and they work out ways to survive in even the most challenging family environments. They evolve strategies to minimise occasions of rejection and maximise their chance of being accepted. They may notice that their parents' behaviour towards them is more accepting when they succeed at school or when they do things to make their parents' lives easier. If they don't 'rock the boat', 'make a fuss' or 'fight back' in some way, they discover that adults – on whom their world depends – seem to treat them better. Because these coping strategies work, at least some of the time, they turn into personal rules to live by.

For example, if a child has been repeatedly put down and hurt by an unresponsive or harshly critical parent, they may devote a lot of energy to making sure that they are liked and approved of by others. A survival 'rule' forms in their mind and they tell themselves that, 'To be accepted, I must make sure I'm liked by other people' or 'In order to be accepted and loved, I must always put others' needs first.' They stop asking for what they really need and they do whatever it takes to please others and to win their approval.

They may notice that achievement buys them acceptance and praise and, as a result, they may adopt a rule of living that says, 'To feel good about myself, I must perform perfectly and always be on top of things.' They learn that to survive, they have to keep a lid on their real feelings and pretend everything is 'just fine'.

It is perfectly natural for human beings to try to stick to

patterns of behaviour where they feel secure – we all want to feel we belong, and we all want to feel good about ourselves – but while these coping strategies or 'rules of living' may work at home and in school when we are young, they do not work well when we become adults. In childhood, we are relatively restricted in our activities, whereas when we become adults, we encounter a much greater range of situations and we need to be flexible rather than rigid if we are to adapt and survive.

Recovery from depression happens when we recognise that many of our 'rules for living' do not work for us any more. We realise that these were the best strategies that we could come up with as children to survive in a difficult situation, but that's it is OK to let them go. We learn to be gentle with ourselves. We recognise that what we need now is to believe in ourselves and try to speak honestly with our own voice, rather than to live for others' approval by avoiding conflict at all costs. Rather than trying to control everything and everyone, we begin to be open and more assertive in our dealings with people.

Of course we don't change overnight; recovery, as outlined in the following chapters, is a path and not some switch we click to make us better. It will bring us moments of great insight and liberation, but there will also be setbacks and moments of terror. The greatest difficulty we face is when we let go of the story we have been telling ourselves all our lives about how we should behave, and when we risk doing something new and different. This is hard because we can be reluctant to let go of the rules that have helped us feel to safe in the world. Without these rules, we are unsure about how to behave and how to manage our relationships.

According to psychoanalyst Donald Winnicott, depression is a state that gives us the time to become aware of – and to choose to change – how we relate to the world. Depression can serve a purpose in that it enables us to slow down and look at what is really hurting us. A positive consequence of depression is that we can achieve a greater level of personal understanding, integration and, ultimately, happiness.

> To our surprise, a person may come out of depression stronger, wiser and more stable than before he or she went into it.
>
> Donald Winnicott, *The Value of Depression*

Social circumstances that cause depression

Sometimes it is not what happened in a person's early life, but rather what is happening in their lives right now that leaves them vulnerable to depression. Poor housing, social isolation and the pressures of rearing young children with no support may be what causes or contributes to a person's depression. One important piece of research, which highlights the crucial role of social support in staying mentally well, is the finding that women in stressful social circumstances with even one close, confiding friend were four times less likely to become depressed, than women in similar circumstances who did not have such a friendship. We all need friendship to lighten the burdens we carry, to restore our trust in ourselves when we lose it, and to break the grip of loneliness that can so easily overtake us when we become isolated.

Regular employment in a job that gives us personal satisfaction gives us a measure of control over our lives and offers numerous opportunities for satisfying interaction with others. Unemployment can leave someone without a regular social support system vulnerable and can also deny them opportunities where they feel they are making some valued contribution. Unemployment can undermine a person's self-confidence and where there is any vulnerability to depression, it may aggravate it.

Research has found that people are 10 times more likely to be depressed if they are unemployed; in other words, being employed decreases one's chance of becoming depressed by a factor of 10.

Many different forms of social injustice exist that can take away a person's dignity. The experience of repeatedly trying, in vain, to deal with an unjust situation can eventually produce what psychologist Seligman called 'learned helplessness'. This is a state of mind where a person loses all confidence in themselves to solve problems in their life, because of having tried repeatedly and having failed to do so. Faced with stress that never seems to go away, and over which a person feels they have little or no control, their confidence to face everyday problems that are normally well within their capabilities becomes worn down. Seligman felt that this state of mind was a key feature of depression. The experience of being bullied and not being able to do anything to stop it is one example of an injustice that can lead to a feeling of helplessness and depression.

Physical factors that cause depression

Whenever we talk about depression, there is a danger of thinking about it exclusively in terms of psychological experiences that cause us hurt. We can forget that we are physical beings with bodies that have a significant impact on how we feel. Some people carry in their bodies a tendency to become depressed, simply because of the constitution they have inherited.

Depression is a very physical experience. Taking care of our bodies is critical to recovery. Medication can be very important for some people, particularly when they are severely depressed or when they have a known vulnerability to bipolar disorder. Exercise and the right kind of nourishment are also critical to both our physical and psychological wellbeing. When we deprive our bodies of these needs, we aggravate the experience of depression. Recovery involves listening to what our bodies need and doing right by them.

Depression is often treated with medication to regulate specific biochemical changes in the brain that are believed to play a part in keeping our mood in a depressed state. Research is not clear what exactly these changes are, but attention has been focused particularly on the role of chemicals that are involved with regulating our emotions. Serotonin is a neurotransmitter that has received particular attention. Antidepressants work by increasing the availability of these chemicals in the brain. In severe episodes of depression, there is believed to be a reduction in the amount of serotonin available in the brain which, in turn, causes fatigue, listlessness and sleep disturbance, so characteristic of depression. Modern antidepressants, called selective serotonin reuptake inhibitors (SSRI), work by increasing the availability of certain chemicals associated with a good mood.

Two broad theories are suggested to account for why a person's brain chemistry may become altered in depression: these are the *genetic* and the *evolutionary* theories.

Genetic theory of depression

The genetic view proposes that some individuals are constitutionally more inclined to become depressed because of a genetic sensitivity they have inherited. Our genes control those chemical processes that occur in the brain, and it is possible that a malfunction in the way key neurochemicals are produced, leads to an individual becoming depressed. Antidepressants are believed to correct this malfunction and their success is often cited as evidence to support this genetic theory.

If it is true that our genetic make-up can cause depression, it should be the case that people with a similar genetic make-up should be equally prone to depression. To investigate this, researchers have focused carefully on the experience of identical twins. According to the genetic explanation for depression, it would be expected that where one twin becomes depressed, the other should too. The evidence from research is that this is broadly the case, with 50 per cent of identical twins likely to become depressed, if the other twin is diagnosed with this problem. This is much more than one would expect in the general population and suggests that there may well be genetic factors at work in depression. However, what is also striking is that many people whose family history might suggest they are at risk for depression do not become depressed. While genetics may render some people more susceptible to depression, many additional factors are likely to be involved in converting a genetic sensitivity to an actual episode of clinical depression.

Evolutionary theory and the 'depressed brain'

In his book *Overcoming Depression*, Professor Paul Gilbert looks to evolutionary theory to account for why everyone is at some level prone to reacting to stress by becoming depressed. His basic idea is that our survival as a species has depended on our capacity to switch into certain brain states if circumstances require it. Thus we have an innate tendency to become anxious in situations where we feel threatened in any way. This is not something we have to think about consciously, it happens automatically as the brain readies the body to cope with danger. The body automatically secretes adrenaline to focus our attention on a possible danger and to energise us to take evasive action.

In the same way, there are also situations that may trigger an innate 'depressive response'. Instead of preparing us by secreting adrenaline to cope with danger, the brain switches into a state where we experience low energy, low mood and a tendency to withdraw into ourselves. This 'depressive response' is activated in situations where we experience the loss of a loved one, and in certain situations where we feel trapped for an extended period of time without any sense that we can escape. As Paul Gilbert describes: 'If we are in unhappy marriages or terrible jobs or live in a place that we hate but can't get away from, we can come to feel that we are stuck, with no way out.'

Another way that the 'depressive response' can be activated is when we demand perfection of ourselves and constantly aim too high in our aspirations. Since the expectations we put on ourselves can never be achieved, we constantly feel a sense of failure and defeat. The brain's response is a way to help us let go of what's not working and refocus our energies in a more productive direction.

Biological factors are very likely to be part of depression for someone with bipolar disorder – a mood disorder where experiences of elation, extreme motor activity, impulsiveness and excessively rapid speech can alternate, or be associated with, severe episodes of depression, as described above. The benefit that specific medications bring to these individuals generally makes them a key element in their recovery.

Summary

Depression can result when we react to sorrow and setbacks by blaming ourselves for the way we feel. Often the reason we do this is that we have carried within ourselves, throughout our lives, a deep insecurity about how loveable and capable we are. When things go wrong in our lives for any reason, we jump to the conclusion that it's 'our own fault'. We imagine that if we could just work harder at being perfect, at pleasing people and keeping a tight control on our inner lives, we would not feel depressed. We can get so used to reacting this way that it's hard to give ourselves a break and accept that our depression may be trying to draw our attention to a part of us that needs healing.

Poor nutrition, lack of exercise or something we have inherited in our physical make-up can also leave us vulnerable to depression.

Sometimes depression has far less to do with our history or with anything inside us, than with our interactions with the world around us. We may be in a difficult relationship that is draining our energies. We may have to cope with an unrelenting bully in our work environment that is completely undermining our self-confidence. Stressful social circumstances where we feel trapped can easily wear us down and leave us vulnerable to depression.

For most of us, it is some combination of the above factors that cause depression. To overcome depression, we need to consider our psychological, physical and social lives in a systematic way. Recovery takes time and we need to be realistic in our expectations and accept that the only place to begin is exactly the place we find ourselves in at this moment in time.

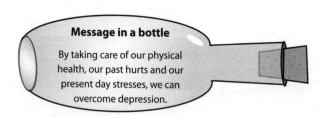

Message in a bottle

By taking care of our physical health, our past hurts and our present day stresses, we can overcome depression.

PART TWO

Recovering from Depression

CHAPTER 3

Taking action to relieve your mood

D epression can be a paralysing experience. You may feel too tired, too alone, too afraid and too confused to see a way out of the prison in which you find yourself. The problem is that your low mood makes it really hard to think clearly and see solutions. Understandably, you may try to distract yourself in various ways – your fingers may roam over the remote control; you log on to the internet and try to lose yourself in a parallel universe; you may eat too much, drink too much; or take to your bed to escape reality.

Whatever relief you get usually only lasts a short time. Very soon you're back ruminating about how pathetic you are for getting into the mess you're in. Your mood feels dark and heavy again. Negative thoughts swarm around inside your head. People around you may offer good advice but nothing they say seems to get through to you. You want to stay put and do nothing, because you are convinced that to try to do anything would only make things worse. In fact, nothing could be further from the truth.

You need a plan of action, something that is not too complicated or too difficult, a plan that will give your day some structure and show you that you can make a difference. This chapter describes three different ways to put you on the road to recovery.

- **Step one** will help you to get your feet moving again. By showing you how to set realistic goals and achieve them, you will discover that it is possible to do something that makes a difference to the way you feel. We are not talking about some amazing transformation of your mood, but something small that you can do that may relieve it even a little and help you to regain your self-confidence. When you become depressed, you can feel like you have lost all control over your life. Small successes rebuild your sense of being in control.

- **Step two** will show you how you can connect with others and find the support you need to get your life back on track.
- **Step three** will show you a simple way to reflect each day on what made a difference to your mood, for better or for worse. Making a habit of writing a few words about the ups and downs you experience each day helps you to see what helps to lift your mood and what brings you down.

Taking responsibility for one day at a time, even one hour at a time, is as much as you can manage at this stage – and each day you do this will bring you one step closer to recovery. As your mood lifts, you will find it easier to confront the problems that got you into a bad mood. Don't try to sort everything out in one go, focus on what you can do and let go of the rest for now.

Step one: Putting some structure back into your life

One of the most consistent findings in the studies on depression is that *activity helps our moods*. Because you may not *feel* like doing anything when you are depressed, it is a good idea to think about one or two things you would like to get done each day and plan how and when you're going to do them. Writing down these activities in a daily diary first thing in the morning (or the night before), focuses your mind on the day ahead. This way you are able to consider doing something that might help your mood, rather than allowing your mood to drag you deeper and deeper into a black hole.

The simple Activity Diary that I've included below has an outline of the day taking one hour at a time and will help you to think about and plan your day, one hour at a time. Alternatively, you may wish to use your own personal notebook or a recovery journal and that's also fine.

When you pick some things to do, don't aim too high; pick tasks that you can manage to complete within the next 24 hours. Plan to do at least one thing that will give you a sense of accomplishment and at least one thing that might be relaxing. A word or two is all that's necessary to describe any activity, e.g. 'breakfast', 'walk', 'clean desk', 'visit friend', 'watch favourite TV programme'.

Nothing succeeds like success when you are depressed. If you set yourself some goals today and complete them, particularly one or two activities that give you a sense of accomplishment, you will most likely feel better able to face tomorrow.

Activity Diary

For each hour slot, write down what activity you did and describe how you felt during that time. Rate how strong these feelings were on a scale of 1 to 10.

Time	Activity	Feelings
9–10 a.m.	Breakfast	Sad, Lonely, (4,5)
10–11 a.m.		
11–12 a.m.		
12–1 p.m.		
1–2 p.m.		

2–3 p.m.

3–4 p.m.

4–5 p.m.

5–6 p.m.

6–7 p.m.

7–8 p.m.

8–9 p.m.

9–10 p.m.

11–12 p.m.

Track your mood

There is something you can add to this exercise that may make it even more interesting for you. Make a note about what you actually do each hour of the day and write down how you felt during that hour beside it. So between 11 and 12 in the morning, you might write 'Went to shop to buy bread' and beside it, in the 'how I felt' column, write whatever you were feeling, for example 'frightened'. If you had different feelings, write as many of them down as you can in the space provided.

Rating how strong your feelings were
Finally, to record how strong your feelings were during each hour, rate this on a scale of 1 to 10 (1=very little; 10=very strong) in your diary as you go through the day, and write down a number beside each feeling.

To summarise, there are two different parts to tracking what you did each day and how you felt:

•   At the beginning of each day, or the night before, write in your

diary two or more activities that are likely to give you a feeling of accomplishment or fun.
- For every hour of the day, describe how you felt, and rate how strong each feeling was, on a scale of 1 to 10.

Think in terms of small steps

A common problem that people who are depressed report is the feeling that they are overwhelmed by the demands on them. There seems to be so much to do, that they feel they can't get a grip on their lives.

Sometimes, your life may seem overwhelming because you're thinking about all of the things you need to do, rather than what you can actually do today. When you think of all the things in your life that need your attention, you feel overwhelmed. When you actually write down the specific things that require your attention today, or in the next few hours, you reduce this feeling. This is a simple idea that is surprisingly powerful when you do it.

Try this for yourself. Make a list of the different stresses that you are facing; decide which you can ignore for the time being and which need your immediate attention.

When you have completed this exercise, consider how much time you will need to complete each task and what would make it easier for you to approach this task. If, for example, you want to write a letter, it might be important to make a time to do this, when interruptions are minimised and when you have time to think about what you want to say. Give yourself plenty of time to complete the task. For example, if you think that writing a letter should only take you an hour, give yourself two or three hours. And consider breaking up the task into small amounts of time, e.g. 30-minute intervals, rather than pushing yourself to get it all done in one go. Our ability to concentrate is reduced when we are depressed and you will very likely find your mind wanders after a relatively short period.

The key to success is to set goals that are achievable. For example, if you would like to exercise and feel that you should walk or run for *at least* three miles a day, you may be setting yourself up for failure. However, if you were to start from where you are – which may be a place where you haven't exercised for months – and set yourself a goal of walking for 10 to 20 minutes a day, you are more likely to succeed and discover through this exercise that you can make a difference to the way you feel.

It is easy to turn up your nose at modest goals. Your pride may insist that you should be able to aim higher. When you aim for something that's possible, every success you experience helps to restore your morale, break the cycle of procrastination and hopelessness, recover the confidence to take on some other things in your life that you have been avoiding and worrying about. Nothing succeeds like success to rebuild hope.

Simplify your life

One thing that may help is to look at your life and see if you've allowed the way you live to become too complicated. Are you trying to live your life on too many fronts? When you're working too hard at trying to do too much, your energies can become depleted and there may be no space in your life to heal and recover.

Sometimes, very simple actions can make a big difference. Dropping some activities that are not essential, taking time to walk and rest, choosing to postpone certain projects that do not require immediate attention, and dealing with something you've been putting off can relieve the pressure you are under. Arranging to take time off and asking for help where you need it most in your life can do the same. Eating well and exercising 30 minutes a day may be as important to your recovery as the time you devote to addressing the deeper roots of your depression.

Don't wait until you 'feel' like doing something

Research has shown that when we are depressed, we react to our distress in the following way: we focus our attention on how we are *feeling*, rather than on what we could *do* to ease our pain. We tell ourselves that, 'If I don't *feel* I can do it, it probably means I shouldn't even try.' We procrastinate and convince ourselves that, 'I'll do it later, when I *feel* more like doing it.'

The problem with this way of thinking is that it assumes that the feeling or *motivation* for doing something should come before you actually do anything. In fact, the opposite is true when you are depressed. Activation precedes motivation. When you feel low, the motivation to do anything comes *after* you've started into the task. If you set about doing something that you've been avoiding and take even very small steps towards achieving your goal, you will be surprised at how the energy for that task does come in the doing of it.

Learn from your activity diary

After you have been keeping an Activity Diary for a few days, you may notice certain patterns that were not clear to you before. You may discover, for example, that your mood is not stuck in one place all the time; that it varies throughout the day, and that what you do makes a difference to the way you feel. Perhaps you can ease your pain by moving towards certain kinds of activities that lift your mood, and by letting go of other activities that seem to get you down.

If the research is right, you should discover that when you are active, your negative mood lightens in intensity. Your depression may not disappear when you do something that gives you a feeling of success or satisfaction, but you may well notice that you don't feel quite as depressed as when you stayed in bed to hide from the world.

Is this what you found? Did you find that there were times when you moved from feeling very down during one hour of the day, to feeling much brighter an hour later? What kinds of activities were associated with these positive mood shifts? You might want to make a note of anything that helped in your 'recovery journal', which I will describe later in this chapter.

Here are some things that Tom, aged 43, learned from tracking his moods and rating his emotions on an hourly basis for a full week:

- My really bad times were in the evenings when I sat in the living-room chair and appeared, to my family, to doze off. In fact I was not sleeping, but withdrawing from everyone.
- When I let my mood sink into a dark place, I found it stayed that way for hours.
- The times I felt best were times when I walked my two racing dogs, and also those times when I felt I had made some important contribution at work.
- Exercise in particular seemed to lift my spirits, but I never really wanted to exercise and when I did, it took nearly an hour of walking before the benefits were noticeable.
- Perhaps the most important thing I learned was that action does precede motivation. It was only after starting to do something that I felt any energy and interest in doing it. When you're depressed, it's not at all a good idea to wait around until you feel like doing something. Just do it, the motivation will kick in soon after you start.

Tom had already been depressed for six years when I met him, and from then onwards he begin to track his activities and emotions. We will consider Tom's story in some depth in Chapter 6 and learn about how he worked his way out of a very dark and difficult place in his life.

Something that can help is to plan to do something that you don't usually do – something novel in your day that breaks your normal routine. Maybe something you've been meaning to try but have never quite got around to. You might plan to attend a music concert or a neighbourhood meeting where you could learn what's planned for your area. The point is to consider breaking your usual routine and try out some new behaviour.

What can I do when I feel really down?

- Accept how I am feeling and be gentle with myself.
- Identify two or more activities that could give my day some structure.
- Make sure there is at least one 'fun' activity in my day.
- Do something that I have never tried before.
- Do one thing at a time.
- Do something badly (rather than not at all).

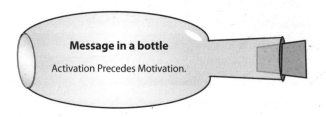

Message in a bottle

Activation Precedes Motivation.

Step two: You don't have to go it alone

Hopelessness thrives when we lose our connection with the world around us. We may feel angry and hurt that life has turned out the way it has and that we have failed in some way. This anger and hurt can turn into bitterness and a stubborn refusal to have anything to do with life.

To overcome depression, you need to move out of isolation and experience genuine contact and nurturing from other people. You won't resolve your depression by trying to figure it out all alone inside your head. Solitude is important at times – it can give you a welcome break and enable you to get some perspective on the problems in your life – but, when you're depressed, solitude can magnify your negative thinking, so that you end up going round and round inside your head without resolving anything.

> Today was a bad day for me, as I couldn't stop worrying about a problem I saw no way to solve. I kept thinking about it, and the more I did, the more I noticed my mood became more depressed. I realised that I needed a break from it all to stop myself slipping into despair. I started by ringing a friend and chatting about something entirely different for 10 minutes. I then took myself out of the house for a short walk. My mood was still 'down' but along the way, I got chatting to some neighbours who were repairing their hall door. They kindly invited me in for tea. Perhaps it was the break, perhaps it was the tea, but I actually feel that it was the human contact that restored my sanity and allowed me let go of my oppressive feelings. I still cared about the problem that remained unresolved, but it no longer consumed me, and I could see possibilities where before I could only see gloom and doom.
>
> John, aged 35

Recovery depends upon you making the choice to help yourself, but that doesn't mean that you have to go it alone. We need contact with other people every day to restore our energy and self-confidence, and to prevent us from becoming isolated and lonely.

Plan to spend some time each day in the company of other people. Sometimes getting support means pausing to chat with somebody you interact with briefly every day, but rarely take time to notice, e.g. the lady in the local shop, the person you buy a train ticket from every morning or the cashier at the supermarket. Even spending a short amount of time with people in a light-hearted way can help to lift your spirits. Perhaps you could visit someone who would welcome some company or make a phone call to an old friend you haven't been in touch with for some time. Or you might pop into a neighbour's house and soak up the atmosphere of warmth and fun that fills their home.

Turning your inner conflicts into a conversation

You don't always need to talk to other people about the way you feel to experience their support, but there are times when it can really help to turn your inner conflict into a conversation with someone who is able to listen.

Recovery from depression involves becoming open to what is troubling you at an emotional level. Painful feelings and associated painful memories often require a safe setting within which you can confide in another person and gain the support you need to talk through what has been avoided for so long. Unwanted feelings and memories are often avoided because people feel they will be too much to bear. The support of a counsellor or friend can enable you to face your fears gradually.

A good listener is someone with whom you feel safe enough to speak, and with whom you can gradually find the words to say what you are feeling. Being able to put your feelings into words enables you to get some distance from how you are feeling and to see more clearly what is happening. When you keep everything bottled up inside, you can't see the wood for the trees and can feel so overwhelmed by all that is happening inside you that you resort to destructive ways to block out and numb your feelings.

Finding someone who can listen intelligently and sensitively can often be difficult. Friends may be supportive and sympathetic but they can only go so far in helping you tease out underlying feelings that may not be very obvious. A qualified psychotherapist who can give you undivided attention can be enormously helpful in making connections between the experiences you have had many years ago and what is troubling you now. A good psychotherapist is someone who will help you to identify practical steps that will relieve your mood and over time, when you are feeling stronger, guide you in exploring some of the root causes of your depression.

Making the decision to talk to someone may be the most difficult step you take, but it may the turning point on your path to recovery. Think about what might work for you. Maybe you have a friend you can trust; or you might check out a support group where there are other people who have been through depression and who understand how you may be feeling; or perhaps what you need most is a professional therapist, to support you and to help you to resolve your depression. The more you can turn your inner conflict into a conversation with others, the greater the chance you have to change how you feel.

Medication: Do I take it or not?

Many of the symptoms of depression are physical in nature. Because of this, many health carers believe that recovery from depression should begin with attempting to change the physical chemistry of the brain. Reduction in the availability of certain neurotransmitters in the brain has been linked to depression and medications are available that regulate the levels of these chemicals specifically and help make recovery a little easier.

Besides the potential benefits of antidepressant medication, there are other physical means of helping to alter your mood and support your recovery. Physical exercise has been found to alter brain chemistry and can enhance mood; good nutrition can be an important element in recovery, particularly because someone who is very depressed can completely overlook the importance of a balanced diet. Finding ways of truly relaxing your body and mind through meditation, aromatherapy, reflexology and sleep, may be key in restoring some level of energy and motivation to face life.

Some people may become uneasy when the option of medication is suggested. They may feel that their problems have been around for a long time and that a deeper focus on their early-life experience may be required if they are to get to the roots of their depression. People often express concern about the possibility of becoming dependent on medication and having to remain on it for the rest of their lives. In addition, the side effects of medication – weight gain and a general feeling of drowsiness – concern many.

Medication can be of great benefit to people with severe depression because it can relieve some of the physical symptoms that characterise depression – exhaustion, lack of energy and sleep disturbance – in a relatively short time. However, medication cannot correct the painful social or emotional factors that have caused depression.

How a doctor addresses the whole issue of medication and recovery is crucial. Sarah, whose journal is featured throughout this book, was fortunate to have a psychiatrist whose view on medication was very realistic. Because she experienced both very deep periods of hopelessness and periods of euphoria, he prescribed medication to help to lift and steady her mood. However, he never gave her the impression that the tablets would sort everything out for her. The way he explained it to her was that medication was only 25 per cent of her recovery. The major part of her recovery was in her own hands – eating correctly, exercising, working through deeper issues in her life in her therapy sessions, finding a job, being active and re-establishing good relationships with her friends and family.

The dogmatism that characterises many professionals working in the field of depression can make it very confusing for people who are trying to work out a recovery plan. Some medical people insist that medication alone will do the job, that the whole reason why a person feels sad is that they have a 'chemical imbalance'. This point of view persists despite the fact that there is, as yet, no specific imbalance that can be identified in people with depression. Initially, this approach may give sufferers a great sense of relief. They are told by a doctor, that what they are feeling is due to a chemical imbalance, and that there is nothing in particular they have to do to get better, other than take medication. The long-term impact of this very narrow view can be very disturbing and confusing for the person concerned. They may feel that the power they had over their lives is no longer theirs, that the medication has taken control. They may come to believe that they have a 'disease' that they can do nothing about, that they are broken and that they can never be fixed.

Equally, there are those who view depression very narrowly as a psychological problem that should be worked out exclusively by long-term psychotherapy. This approach may ignore ways in which the body and the brain influence our mood, thereby denying someone the potential benefit of medication.

What people need when they are feeling depressed, is someone who has their best interests at heart, and who is willing to consider the unique circumstances they are in, someone who has experience of seeing and helping people to recover from depression, and who appreciates the many different ways that people can achieve recovery. People who are depressed need someone who can takes an informed holistic view and not be blinkered by their favourite theory of depression, be it medical or psychological.

The picture is somewhat clearer when you look at the research on effective treatment for depression. Results of numerous studies conclude that some forms of psychotherapy are as effective as medication in reducing mild and moderately severe depression, but that the combination of medication and therapy seems to be more beneficial than either one alone when it comes to severe depression. Psychotherapy has also been found to decrease vulnerability to relapse, while relapse is very likely when medication is discontinued, and when the deeper causes of depression have not been addressed. Medication may be particularly important to consider where the sufferer reports an intense experience of pain, a family history of depression or strong suicidal feelings.

Whatever help you get, remember that no matter how bad you are feeling, this is your life and no one has the right to insist that you adhere to their advice. A good doctor or therapist will always make you aware that you are the person who has to learn from your depression and work through it; that there is no magic pill or therapy that will suddenly make everything right. People may give you lots of advice, and mean well when they do, but at the end of the day, what matters is that you find the path to recovery that is right for you, and that you take small steps to work towards that goal.

Consulting your GP

If you are looking for someone to help you overcome depression try to find someone who appreciates the value of different therapeutic approaches, and who is willing to consider what your particular experience of depression may require in order for you to achieve a full recovery. A good GP is the starting place for most people and generally he or she can advise on medication and arrange a referral to appropriate specialists on your behalf.

If you make an appointment with your GP, there are some things you can do beforehand to help you make the most of your time with him or her. Think about what you are going to say to communicate how you feel. Identify *three* words that describe the way you have been feeling over the past few days or weeks. For example, you may summarise how you have been feeling with the words 'tired', 'alone', 'no energy' – use words and phrases that feel right to you. Tell the doctor how long you have been feeling this way, and, finally, tell them how you are coping with your life and how you are *not* coping.

Keep it simple. Don't allow yourself to become distracted by worries that you are wasting the doctor's time. Expect that when you are in your GP's office, you may have the following thoughts, 'I shouldn't be talking so much about myself' or 'I am wasting the doctor's time'. Many people who seek help and advice for 'emotional' problems worry that their problems are not as important as other people's problems. In fact, you are just as important as anyone else and your doctor appreciates the courage it takes to open up about your problems.

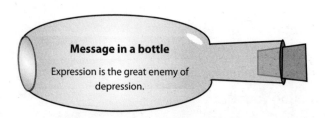

Message in a bottle

Expression is the great enemy of depression.

Step three: Reflecting on each day and learning about what works for you

Recovery takes time. It is important to keep this in mind, to be gentle with yourself, and to be patient with the time that may be required. For some, it can be quite rapid – particularly when an obvious stress in their life is resolved or when medication seems to 'hit the spot' and lift their mood – but for the majority of people who experience depression, recovery can be a matter of two steps forward, one step back. Their mood can lift significantly for a period of time but good days can be followed for a time by gloomy days. Energy that seems to be available for an evening can be curiously absent the next morning.

I remember one man who became quite frustrated with me around the same time that his mood began to lift. During one of our therapy sessions he said:

> In any given week, I have about four good days and three bad ones. The problem is I never can predict how I'll be tomorrow. Before I started therapy, I felt miserable seven days a week, but at least life was predictable!

Below are two diagrams. The first illustrates what people imagine recovery looks like and the other shows what recovery is actually like:

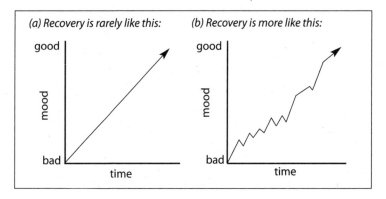

Keeping a recovery journal

Keeping a diary and reflecting on your experience each day can greatly help your recovery. Your mood will vary, but there may be something you can learn from this, if you stand back and look at what kind of things bring you down and what kind of things give you a lift. Maybe there is no obvious pattern to your mood swings, but by keeping track of the changes you may at least be able to see that your mood is fluid and changeable rather than fixed and permanent.

I recommend buying a large notebook and making entries on a daily basis. You may prefer to open a file on your computer, a 'recovery file', and make entries each day. You may write a lot or simply a few words. You may use words or you may prefer to draw images or use colours that reflect your experience.

What you write about will vary, depending on what is important to you on a given day. For example, you may want to write about how badly you are feeling or you may want to make a note about something that helped your mood. You may want to acknowledge something you did that made a difference and give yourself credit for even the smallest successes you experienced. Each step you take in recovery, no matter how small, is significant and worth noting. On the days you feel like writing longer entries, you may consider writing about some early experiences in your life that may have left you vulnerable to depression.

Sarah was attending university when she came for help and she complained of feeling down, being unable to concentrate and withdrawing from friends. Soon after she started therapy, it became clear that her problems were complex and her mood much more depressed than it had initially appeared. Writing down how she was feeling and what she was thinking every day was one of the most important ways in which she worked her way out of depression.

Sarah's recovery journal

Excerpt 4

I want to live. I want to care and I want to love. I want to be capable of failing but not falling apart. And I want warmth.

I want to feel loved and cared for, not neglected and ignored. I want to know and learn how not to neglect and ignore myself. I'd like to be me. By writing this journal and asking to have someone read it, I realise I'm asking to be listened to, to be heard, to be read, to be understood, to be treated as a living person who is hurting so much inside and needs to be cared for and who needs some kind of compassion to help me keep going and discover some way to ground myself. This notebook says more than any verbal discourse because it's a concentrated effort of really writing down how I am. It's true, it's painful and it hurts to do this, but at least I'm now allowing this pain to surface. For most of my life, I've refused to acknowledge my feelings and this has distorted my sense of myself. I've not been able to have any clear sense of who I am but since I've allowed myself to write things down, I've become much clearer about the person that I am inside.

Writing is becoming a comfort to me. It's a space on paper where I can express myself without any judgement at all. It is a sanctuary of hope where I can begin to discover things I do not know about myself. It's a labyrinth of words, thousands upon thousands, which I have needed to relocate a sense of myself. I need to write so much. I have to. It's only when I write that I begin to effectively identify something about the way I feel and in so doing I become more definite about who I am.

Writing about her experience of recovery proved to be very helpful to Sarah. The amount she wrote varied greatly from day to day. Some days she felt incredibly despondent, and on others there was evidence of hope and strength returning.

For some people, writing may not come so easily. This is certainly the case when depression is felt intensely. You can't concentrate enough to write, your mind wanders and you find yourself getting caught up in negative ruminations over which you have little control. During these times, the emphasis in your recovery has to be on *doing* things that bring relief. Take a walk, listen to or play some music, find a quiet bench in a local park, or if you can, get down to the sea, watch the incoming tide, and let your mind become calmed by the beauty of it all. Later, when your mood has slightly lifted, see if you can write a little about what has been happening for you, and what seems to be helping.

Pay attention to even very tiny breakthroughs

When you feel depressed, you see your whole life through a dark lens. It is more than likely that you filter out everything good that ever happened to you, and remember only those experiences that fit with the painful way you feel in the present. You may not see this 'memory bias' at work, because it happens automatically, without you ever noticing. Writing can be a way to correct this bias and to acknowledge small but significant breakthroughs.

At the end of each day, see if you can recall an event that lifted your spirits. Record these experiences in your journal. Being thankful for moments like these can ease the pain of depression and restore a larger perspective on your life.

You can also learn something important from moments that were particularly difficult. Maybe you bit off more than you could chew at this time. Maybe you need to change your expectations of yourself. Are you asking more of yourself at this time than is realistic? Are you pushing yourself because you think that you have to make up for being so miserable inside? You are struggling with a lot, so credit yourself for making the effort and succeeding to whatever degree you can. As you record moments in the day where you felt badly, consider what it was that upset you. It may have to do with something that someone said or did to you, or it may have been that your drop in mood had more to do with the way you turned against yourself, when this happened. We look more closely at this in Chapter 4.

The excerpt from Sarah's journal below reflects the benefit she gained from attending to some everyday chores and to some homework she'd been putting off. Her comments at the end of this entry reveal questions she was beginning to ask herself concerning her deeper feelings. She explored these issues at a later stage of her recovery, but her mention of them in this entry suggested she was feeling strong enough in herself to at least ask these questions and look at what she was feeling.

Sarah's recovery journal

Excerpt 5

I spent the day in the flat as my cough was quite bad and I didn't feel like going into college to exhaust myself. I had breakfast, watched some TV, ironed and tidied my clothes and then did a translation for homework which took hours. I was happy to have completed this, although I still have to check it for grammar mistakes. Although it took me so long to do this work and I know I have a huge amount of work to catch up with, I don't seem to feel that bad about it. Tonight I feel quite relaxed. I think part of this is because I was alone for most of the day and I got something done which made me feel productive.

I wonder where my feelings are hiding tonight because it's unlike me to write so much factual stuff. I'd love it if one day I were to sit down and put pen to paper producing pages and pages about my feelings. I'd love to unblock parts of me that are so afraid of opening. I wouldn't want to open each little door inside of me, but I want to see the names on those doors and at least see inside some of those rooms. I'd like to know what's there. I'd like to see what's hiding inside. I don't want to always be afraid of holding these feelings back. I want to let them live inside me.

Summary

- Take control of your day, put some structure on the day and be sure to plan to do two activities that are likely to give you a sense of personal accomplishment.
- Spend some time in the company of other people and friends and draw on their warmth.
- Reflect on what you learned from the day. If you can't write much, take some 'time out' in whatever way is most relaxing for you and consider what was most life-giving for you today.
- Remember, it is very hard to get started on any activity when you feel depressed. Be gentle with yourself and give yourself lots of encouragement when you manage to achieve even 'tiny' steps.

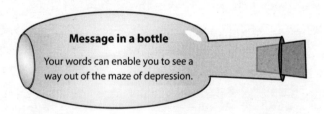

Message in a bottle

Your words can enable you to see a way out of the maze of depression.

CHAPTER 4

Catching your thoughts

P eter was in his twenties with a very promising career. Two years earlier, he had stopped work because of vague symptoms of ill health that were eventually diagnosed as being caused by depression. He'd been unpopular and bullied at school. His reaction to this had been to adopt an attitude of competitiveness to overcome his fear of rejection by his peers. Winning was how he felt he could gain acceptance. And it worked a lot of the time. However, he drove himself relentlessly in every aspect of his life and he took failure very badly. Anything less than perfection made him annoyed with himself to the point where he would verbally attack himself. His constant pushing and berating of himself had clearly contributed to his mental exhaustion. 'My being sick', he said, 'allowed me to avoid killing myself by trying so hard at work. My illness is a sign I need to change my life, to stop listening to my mind and try listening to my body.'

At 17, with the Leaving Certificate successfully behind her and a warm, attractive personality that drew others to her, Jennifer was highly insecure and prone to severe mood slumps. Many of her relatives had experienced chronic depression and this had affected all the children in different ways. But Jennifer was determined to hold on to some semblance of mental health and not succumb to the behaviours she had observed at home. Frequent battles were waged within her mind between the part of her that wanted to break free from home and the part of her that felt guilty that she wasn't doing more to make those around her 'better'. In those periods where she felt down, she would turn against herself with an attitude of self-loathing, picking on details of her appearance – 'I don't look like any kind of life form until I wear make-up' – her intelligence – 'I am so thick' – and her confusion about her future – 'I don't know what to do with my life'. These thoughts would take hold of her mind, driving her mood into intense hopelessness and provoking her to withdraw from friends who could keep her grounded. What looked initially like normal teenage 'angst' soon became a serious mood problem that would last for weeks.

Reading the above accounts of two people who were no strangers to depression, you might be tempted to ask many questions regarding what caused their problems. However, I wonder as you read the above accounts, if you can spot something they both have in common.

Both Peter and Jennifer tried to deal with their vulnerability to depression by driving themselves harder to get on with their lives. They could each sense when their energy was dropping and when they were sinking into a black hole. Rather than trying to suppress their mood, they would try to talk themselves out of it. They would remind themselves how weak they were to be giving in. They used blame and shame to try to pull themselves together. We call this style of reacting 'rumination'. While it may probably be the most common way for humans to try to pull out of a downward spiral, it generally makes things worse. When we ruminate in this way, we actually push ourselves deeper into the very hole from which we are trying to escape.

Research on depression has identified particular patterns of thinking that seem to deepen our depression. Our thinking becomes distorted so that we see our world, our future and ourselves 'through a glass darkly'. We turn on ourselves, heaping self-criticism and self-loathing on the 'pathetic' individual we now believe we are, we see the world around us as unsympathetic and unsupportive, and we view our future as a never-ending continuation of our present painful state of mind. Our gloomy thoughts intensify our feelings of hopelessness, fear and anger. Our behaviour, in turn, reflects our state of mind as we withdraw from other people.

To recover from depression we need to become aware of our thinking, and find some way to calm our minds when it becomes tormented. When the mind settles, we begin to see things more clearly and we can then talk to ourselves in a more compassionate way. Gradually we are able to steady ourselves and we see different possibilities for ourselves. Our hopefullness lifts and we see that the supports we need are all around us.

The link between thoughts and moods

In the past 30 years, cognitive therapy has explored in some depth the kinds of thoughts that intensify depression and how we can loosen our attachment to these thoughts. The word 'cognitive' refers to the way we think, the way we look at things. This approach takes as its guiding principle that it is not so much what happens in our life that determines our moods, but rather how we think about and how we interpret what happens to us. Our emotional reactions, and how we respond to events, depend on the way we think about our lives from one moment to the next.

Aaron Beck, the founder of this therapeutic approach, had

been working at the University of Pennsylvania in Philadelphia in the 1950s as a psychoanalyst when he began to observe certain features among people who were depressed. He noticed that the thoughts that spontaneously passed through their minds in response to any given situation had an immediate impact on how they felt. These thoughts and images – which Beck refers to as 'cognitions' – were characteristically self-blaming and defeatist. The people with whom he was working took any kind of setback very personally, and tended to feel it was their fault entirely.

How we 'read' any given situation can determine how we feel. If we typically blame ourselves for whatever has gone wrong, and regard it as 'all my fault', then we should not be surprised that we feel poorly motivated to deal with that situation. Our thinking can steal away our self-confidence to solve the problems we encounter. So we push ourselves to 'put up' with the situation, to 'stop complaining' about what can't be changed, and we sink deeper and deeper into helplessness.

Discovering new ways of thinking can open up new possibilities for responding creatively to difficult situations. Beck found that by becoming aware of the negative thoughts that accompany our moods, and seeing them as thoughts rather than truths, we can stop ourselves from being carried away by them.

Daily Mood Log

To help you to become aware of your particular self-defeating thinking patterns and to get some distance from them, it is important to write them down. I have included a Daily Mood Log that you can use regularly (page 65) to help you become aware of your negative thinking when you feel upset, and also to discover how these negative thoughts give rise to painful feelings.

Daily Mood Log		
Situation	Feelings	Automatic thoughts

Step one: Describe the situation where you noticed yourself feeling depressed

Consider a recent situation where you became upset and perhaps stayed that way for some time afterwards. Pick a situation that is still fresh in your mind. It doesn't have to be one of the most upsetting events in your life. It's actually easier to pick a mildly upsetting event, rather than something too traumatic, to ease yourself in to this exercise.

Be as specific and as concrete as you can. In column 1 of your Daily Mood Log, under 'Situation', record when it happened, *where* you were, *what* you were doing, *who* you were with, *what* time you became upset. You might write down something like: 'Thursday, 10.05 p.m., alone at home, got a phone call from Barbara, and immediately after noticed I was upset.' Being specific about the precise situation that upset you will help you stay focused throughout this exercise when you attempt to recapture your feelings and thoughts.

Sometimes it's hard to pin point a precise external event that triggered your mood. For example, you might simply be sitting reading the newspaper when you suddenly notice yourself feeling quite low. Nothing that you were reading or that was going on around you seemed to be particularly distressing. This kind of 'out of the blue' experience is very common. The explanation for it will become clearer when you identify what thoughts or images were passing through your mind at the time. For the moment, just make a note of where you were when you started to feel down, and if you can remember being preoccupied with someone or something, add 'thinking about X'.

Step two: Identify the different emotions you felt at the time

To understand your negative reactions to certain situations, it is important to identify as precisely as you can the feelings you had at the time. While you may be very clear that you felt upset, it may take you some time to pin point the different kinds of feelings that were part of that 'upset' experience.

Whereas thoughts are 'mental' events that pass through your mind, feelings are your body's way of reacting. To help you name your feelings, try to remember how your body felt at the time. Where in your body did you notice you were upset? What did this sensation feel like?

If you find yourself becoming confused about the different feelings you had, try to focus on the situation you were in at the time and jot down as many details as you can to describe it. Who else was present? What else was going on around you? For example, John recalled feeling upset at home one evening quite suddenly, and initially he couldn't make any sense of it. When he reflected on what was going on around him at the time, he remembered watching a film that portrayed a mirror image of his own unhappy marriage. A particular scene in this film had reminded him of all the ways he felt he had failed his wife. Identifying and recalling the situation in a detailed way makes it much easier to recapture the different feelings that were triggered.

Listed below are feelings that are very commonly reported by people who feel depressed. See if any of the words listed 'fit' with what you felt at the time on the occasions you were upset. Don't feel limited by this list. Feel free to use any other words that describe uniquely how you felt in such a situation.

List of common negative feelings				
Sad	Anxious	Ashamed	Irritated	Lonely
Depressed	Frightened	Embarrassed	Frustrated	Insecure
Hurt	Nervous	Exposed	Edgy	Abandoned
Hopeless	Agitated	Guilty	Angry	Lost
Heartbroken	Panicky	Humiliated	Mad	Rejected

The most common difficulty experienced in completing a mood log is separating thoughts from feelings. This is because they are so closely connected in our experience. We separate them because it makes it easier for us to see what happens when we get upset, and to identify those places in ourselves where we are most vulnerable. A simple rule of thumb is that feelings are felt in the body and they can generally be described in one word. If it takes more than one word to describe a feeling, it may be that you're describing a thought. Thoughts are the spontaneous words, memories or visual images that pass through our mind when we react to something.

Step three: Identify your automatic thoughts

Column 3 of the mood log invites you to record your 'negative automatic thoughts'. These are the thoughts that pass spontaneously through your mind in response to some event. They are described as 'automatic' because they just happen, without any particular deliberation or reflection on your part. They may take the form of specific statements, such as: 'Oh, God, this is terrible!', 'I can't possibly handle this', 'I'm no good at dealing with this kind of situation', 'It's my own fault, I should have been able to avoid this happening'.

Automatic thoughts may also take the form of fleeting images or fragments of memories that are triggered in a particular situation. It can take time for us to identify what exactly passed through our minds when we became upset but, when we do, it helps us to make sense of our reactions and this helps us to feel less bewildered, less weird and more in control.

Recovery from depression for Sarah involved keeping a record of her thoughts and moods and gradually learning to talk back to them. The following journal entry describes what she discovered on one occasion during her hospitalisation when she became upset. It happened during one of our therapy sessions when she realised she was really thirsty and needed a drink. The particular medication she was taking had made her mouth very dry and it was becoming difficult for her to keep talking. However, she was afraid to ask if she could leave to get some water and sat for 30 minutes in session before admitting her need. When eventually she did ask to leave for a moment, she stood up and exclaimed, 'My God, I've actually asked for something!' It was a significant moment for her and I asked her to make a note of her thoughts and feelings as she sat for those 30 minutes, afraid to make her request. This is what she wrote.

Sarah's recovery journal		
Excerpt 6		
Situation	Feelings	Automatic thoughts
Tuesday, 12.30 p.m. During therapy session with TB. I wanted to leave the session for a moment to get a drink of water, but I was too afraid to ask.	Scared Ashamed Selfish Insecure	I'm annoying somebody when I don't really need to. I'm being demanding. TB will resent me for not anticipating that I'd need water during the session. He'll think I'm stupid. He'll see me as worthless and not want to work with me any more. If I ask for what I need, I may lose whatever little I'm getting.

In completing this exercise, Sarah was surprised to discover that the many different feelings she felt were directly related to the thoughts that she was having at the time. Writing these down made her feel better because her experience of feeling upset now made sense to her. It was not surprising that she felt 'scared' when she realised that she was frightened that I would react negatively to her wanting a drink and that, in her mind, I would not take her seriously. Writing down her thoughts also revealed one of her deeper beliefs about herself that had an enormous influence on the way she related to others – 'If I ask for what I need, I may lose whatever little I'm getting.' Through this exercise, we were able to focus on this belief and we looked at all the ways it had shaped her dealings with the hospital staff, i.e. not talking much to the staff, always seeming to be in good form even when she was miserable and her apparent indifference to nurses when they asked if she needed anything.

Attending to negative thinking is an important aspect of recovery because you learn to begin to catch these thoughts at an early stage before your mood slumps into a dark place. When you see how powerfully they affect your mood and how they undermine your self-confidence to act in a constructive way, you are less inclined to automatically 'buy in' to them. By writing down the negative thoughts associated with your depression, you start to recognise that you keep having the same thoughts over and over again. There may be no more that five or six key negative thoughts that pass through your mind 'automatically' every time you start to feel depressed.

Where do they come from? Why do they keep coming back? Most likely they originate from a time in our life when blaming yourself and pushing yourself seemed like the only way you could survive a difficult situation.

The antidote to these negative thoughts and beliefs is not to force yourself to 'think positively'. Before you can think about the challenges and setbacks you encounter in a more constructive way, you first need to thank these negative thoughts for the way they have been trying to protect you all your life. Even if believing them has caused you pain, you need to recognise that their function was to try to save you from even greater pain. The negative thinking patterns were the best you could do when all you had to work with was the mind of a child, and you felt threatened by the world around you. But now it is time to let them go and to draw on your adult intelligence to think in a kinder and more creative way about the difficulties that you face.

Changing how you think

Let's look more closely at these negative thought patterns and see if we can identify what exactly it is about them that makes them not just unhelpful, but untrue. A longer version of the Daily Mood Log (page 76) will help you finds ways to 'talk back' to your negative thoughts and think about your life in a different way.

As you read over Sarah's thoughts, you may notice certain characteristics they have in common with your own when you become upset. They always place you in the worst light possible, e.g. 'I'm annoying somebody ... I'm being demanding', they usually assume the worst as far as other people are concerned, e.g. 'He'll think I'm stupid', and they present a picture of the world where things will almost certainly get worse, e.g. 'He'll see me as worthless and not want to work with me any more'.

There are some specific ways that negative thinking can undermine your mood. Each of these negative thought patterns has a particular sting to it that distorts your thinking so that you always see things in the worst possible way. Beck has identified a number of different ways in which our thinking can lead us into blind alleys. The 'cognitive distortions' he identified are described in detail by David Burns in *The Feeling Good Handbook* and by Paul Gilbert in *Overcoming Depression*. Below are some examples of the most common ways our thinking trips us up when we become depressed.

1. **Personalisation:** This is where we blame and criticise ourselves relentlessly and take everything bad that happens personally. When we do this, we are assuming a degree of control over life and other people that is completely unrealistic.
2. **Mind-reading:** We assume that we can read the minds of others and we imagine others are being as rejecting of us as we are of ourselves.

3. **All or nothing thinking**: We demand perfection from ourselves and we regard anything less as complete failure. We are completely unforgiving of ourselves and insist that we should be able to be strong and capable all of the time.
4. **Over generalisation**: We interpret one setback, or one bad day, as a sign of endless defeat.
5. **Discounting the positive**: We disregard the good things we have done on any one day and dwell on what didn't work out.
6. **Catastrophisation**: We frighten ourselves by thinking of the very *worst* that could happen rather than anything positive that could happen.

Below is an example of an exercise which Ann, a student nurse, completed one week before her final exams when she felt upset and unable to concentrate. She identified her negative thoughts and the main distortions that characterised these thoughts. This gave her enough relief and clarity of mind to think about her situation in a more helpful way, and to focus on her work.

Ann's Mood Log		
• Feeling stresssed before an exam		
Negative thoughts	**Distortion**	**More helpful response**
I shouldn't feel this way	All or nothing	It would be nice if I felt better, but feeling stressed before exams is not surprising. Being ashamed and resentful of my feelings only adds to my problems.
I'm stupid, I always make mistakes	Discounting the positive	I'm human, not stupid; and 'even I' make mistakes! I also have

		done some things really well on this course.
I have too much to do – I can't manage – I'll mess up this exam and never finish this course	Catastrophising	I'm just frightening myself by thinking this way. I'd do a lot better to write out what I can achieve today and get on with it.

Below are some ways to help you challenge your negative thinking.

Ask yourself, 'What would I say to a good friend in a similar situation?' or 'Would I be as critical towards them as I am to myself?' You might also find it helpful to consider what a good friend might say to you if you described the situation where you became distressed and overwhelmed. Can you picture them there beside you being encouraging and supportive? What are they saying to you? How are they saying it?

Generally when we think in distorted ways, we leap to some conclusion without having any evidence that it is true. For example, we mind-read what others are thinking and imagine that they are being severely critical of us without ever actually asking them whether or not we did something to annoy or upset them. The key to breaking the grip of our negative thoughts is to learn to stand back from them and to ask ourselves, 'Is this really true or am I just reacting to this situation in the way that I have always tended to react to situations like this?'

Recovery from depression is about gradually learning to think and act in ways that build your self-confidence and about not allowing yourself to be bullied into helplessness and defeatism by negative thinking. This takes practise and you will notice how easy it is at times to slip into old habits. But that's because you've been thinking in a certain way all your life until now. These thoughts will never go away entirely. What does change is that you begin to see them for what they are and let them be, without buying into them. Negative thoughts may reappear from time to time but you won't believe in them any more. You recognise that while they may have been the best you could do at one time in your life, they seriously undermined your self-confidence. Recovery takes hold when you decide you want to choose how you want to live your life.

Gradually, you learn to *become kinder to yourself.* You will learn to be encouraging of your efforts to cope with life.

> I'm doing OK, this isn't easy for me but I'm hanging in, I'm getting there.

You stop and *check things out.*

> What can I do to check if this is really true before I get myself all worked up about it?

If something goes wrong, you *don't assume it's your fault entirely.*

> OK, so this didn't quite work. But maybe it wasn't all my fault. What are the different things that could have contributed to this not working out?

You stop assuming that you can read minds, and you *ask others what they think.*

> I actually don't know how Mary feels about my being depressed. Maybe I could ask her and find out?

Summary

- How you think about your life determines how you feel.
- When you are depressed, your thinking becomes negative and distorted.
- Negative thinking lowers your self-esteem, makes you less trusting of others and makes it hard for you to deal effectively with challenges you face.
- It is possible to become aware of particular negative thoughts that upset you, and to learn to think about your life in a more open, creative way.
- As you learn to think about yourself in a kinder and more encouraging way, your self-confidence will rise and you will see that for every problem you face, there is a solution.

Self-help exercise

You can change the way you think. The most important thing is to become aware of what's happening when you feel upset. The short form of the Daily Mood Log can help you to sharpen your awareness. The longer form will help you to change your reactions to everyday challenges and setbacks. As you practise writing out your thoughts and talking back to them, you will find that it is possible to do this very quickly in your head when you notice yourself becoming upset.

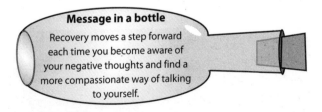

Message in a bottle
Recovery moves a step forward each time you become aware of your negative thoughts and find a more compassionate way of talking to yourself.

Daily Mood Log (Extended Version)			
Situation	Feelings	Negative automatic thoughts	Alternative, more helpful ways of thinking

Key questions to help you construct an alternative response to a negative thought.

1. What would you say to a friend who was in the same predicament? What might a friend say to you?
2. Do you really know this is true? Could there be some way you could check the evidence?
3. Can you see any way in which your thinking may be distorted?
4. What would be a fairer and more helpful way of thinking?

CHAPTER 5

Changing your self-image

Your self-image is the sum total of all that you believe about the kind of person you are: what you are capable of; how loveable you are; what you have in you to give to the world. When your self-image is positive, you believe in yourself, you have an inner confidence that you can solve problems, and when you meet a challenge that is too much for you, you are not afraid to ask for help. You know your strengths, you accept your limitations, and you set goals that are realistic and attainable.

People who are vulnerable to depression generally have a poor self-image. Perhaps as a result of particular negative childhood experiences, they doubt that they are 'lovable' and 'capable'. Depression is sparked when these self-doubts are activated. When something happens that sets off a person's worst fears, they feel all the same painful feelings that they experienced, when their self-image was originally wounded. If they were mistreated as a small child, a rejection in their adult life can trigger all the feelings of hurt and loneliness they felt at that time. If they were bullied in school, the wound of humiliation they experienced as a child can be reopened in their later life by the slightest criticism. When old wounds are opened, a person's belief that there is something 'wrong' with them can be reinforced. They become depressed because they lose faith in themselves; their depression, in turn, seems to prove that all their doubts about themselves must be true, that they are fundamentally flawed and that nothing can change that.

It might not be at all obvious that people have a very low opinion of themselves. When a person believes they are lacking in some way, they may try hard to behave in a way that makes them 'acceptable' to others. They cultivate a 'survival' personality and do whatever they can to keep their imagined flaws hidden from others. Like all of us, they want to be accepted and to belong with other people.

If a person has heard repeatedly as a child that they were 'bad' for whatever reason, they may make a strenuous effort to be 'good', to do 'the right thing'. If they learned that being 'dependent' or emotionally needy was unacceptable, they may try hard to disown their own emotional needs, and act like they are 'independent' and 'self-reliant'. If they believe that their feelings 'don't matter', they may content themselves with looking after everyone else rather than ever asking for what they themselves need.

A positive self-image is the best protection we have against recurrent depression. Any recovery plan has to consider ways to give someone the opportunity to heal their self-image. But the beliefs that make up a negative self-image are formed in early life, and they can feel absolutely true. Changing them may well be the hardest work that someone will ever have to do in their lives.

These underlying doubts and fears usually become the focus of psychotherapy after a person has recovered from the more intense symptoms of their depression. A person needs to feel strong before they can stand back and see that the image they formed of themselves in early life was not at all a true image of who they really are. While it may be liberating to discover that much of what they learned about the kind of person they are is not true, letting go of these false beliefs and finding a new identity can feel very disruptive. But this work is fundamental to making a lasting recovery from depression. This chapter will describe some of the ways this can happen.

I am a rock

If you have never felt loved for just being yourself, you may do whatever you imagine it takes to achieve a sense of belonging with others. Alternatively, you may try to convince yourself that other people's acceptance doesn't matter and go it alone. You act independently, rely completely on yourself and invest yourself in your work. You may feel starved of real intimacy and affection, but you keep your distress hidden, until the pain of chronic loneliness gives way to depression.

By his mid-forties, Richard had set up his own company and developed it successfully over a number of years. He was single and had never been able to establish a close bond with anyone. He had suffered a number of bouts of depression in his life following the death of a close sibling but he had never spoken about the effect this loss had had on him. He relied on 'self-medicating' himself with alcohol to get through his black periods.

In spite of his inner torment, he managed to 'keep up appearances', because he had grown up believing that if he showed weakness of any kind, other people would despise him. This was a belief he had 'come by honestly' at home, where his parents had always viewed with contempt people who were in any way vulnerable.

After several episodes of depression, Richard began to feel too exhausted to go it alone any more. Late one evening, he came to a clear decision that he would end his suffering once and for all. He took a can of petrol to an isolated location and, in the early hours of a bleak morning, sat in his car and set it on fire. By a sheer coincidence, a farmer was passing in a nearby field, spotted the rising smoke and came to Richard's assistance. Richard was rushed to a local Burns Unit and spent several months recovering, both physically and emotionally.

No one in his life had had any idea that he had been in such despair, until he spoke to them about how he had been living 'two parallel lives' – one where he was social and competent in his interactions with others; the other where he felt isolated and alone. When he was first resuscitated in hospital, he was not pleased. But this changed when he was able to be honest for the first time about his experience with his siblings and friends, and he discovered that they were more accepting and supportive than he had ever imagined possible.

When Richard was close to discharge and had worked through many of the issues that had distressed him, he said that he was grateful in many ways for the fire because it had 'burned away' the façade of his social personality, which had only served to cut him off from others all his life. The fire exposed what was inside him to others and he experienced their love and support, which had been unavailable to him for all of his life because of his self-imposed isolation.

Each of us to some extent lives two lives, an inner emotional life and an outer social life. It is important that we can exercise our personal boundaries and keep certain things to ourselves. Privacy is one of our rights and it is important that we know this. However, when the gap between our inner life and our outer life becomes too great, we sense a strain. This is an important warning sign that something is not quite right.

Excessive secrecy can lead to a breakdown of communication between our inner world and the world around us. We deprive ourselves of the vital nurturing we need from others. When we lack a genuine connection with other people, we can begin to feel as if we are dying inside. We feel we are no longer living but simply existing. The masks we wear hide our pain, but they also cut us off from any opportunity to heal.

A therapeutic relationship with someone with whom we feel safe can be a crucial step for restoring a channel of communication between our inner experience and other people. It can enable us to recover our own voice and speak our truth. As we slowly find the words to tell another person how we really feel, we ease back the curtains we've drawn around ourselves. Shafts of light enter our inner world. At first the light hurts our eyes but gradually we see colour and texture where before was only dreary monotony.

Communication enables us to see clearly the fears and self-doubts that have plagued us for years. We see how we have put so much of our energies into hiding from others and we realise how self-defeating this has been. We begin to understand where and when we learned to live so defensively and to see that we don't have to keep doing this if we choose not to. We discover in ourselves that we can communicate in an open way and that when we do, other people are able to support us.

As we change these patterns, we make new choices that alter the course of our lives. A relationship with a therapist can be one way of finding the clarity and inner strength to move from mistrust to trust. Initially, this can feel extremely frightening because we feel so vulnerable without our usual defences, but, over time, the experience of being open enables us to become strong and helps us to feel alive.

What can we learn from Richard's story?

- Excessive secrecy and shame lead to isolation and loneliness.
- Isolation is fertile soil for the seeds of depression.
- Finding someone we can trust can open our minds to seeing life in a new way.

> - Never underestimate the support that people can and will give you if you take the risk of asking.
> - Opening up to the world around us takes courage.

My needs don't matter, other people are more important than me

Some people build their self-image around the belief that says, 'What I want is not important, what others expect of me is the only thing that matters.' They regard this as 100 per cent true and never think to question it. Their lives become a matter of constantly watching others, and trying to live up to what they imagine others expect of them.

There are a number of childhood experiences that set a person up for behaving in this way. A child may experience that it is only when they do something to makes their parents happy, that they are noticed and praised. They learn that to be loved, they must take care of others, rather than seek to be cared for. They grow up with an acute sensitivity to the needs of those around them and they feel compelled to 'look after' everyone. They may become compulsive carers, applauded for their endless generosity and readiness to help.

However, this pattern of over caring for others and disowning one's personal needs can leave a person vulnerable to feelings of exhaustion and resentment. At some point, the inner build-up of frustration may explode, much to the shock of family, friends and co-workers who have never realised that this person needed as much love and care as they had been showing others. Mental health is about finding a way of relating to others that is based on 'give and take'. Too much giving leaves us vulnerable to depression.

Fear lurks behind a compulsive need to care. Sarah described how she had always felt afraid of causing upset in her childhood, and subsequently became overly concerned with looking after the needs of others and disowning her own needs. In Chapter 4, we noted some of Sarah's negative thoughts associated with her fear of asking for a drink of water during her therapy session. Subsequently, we explored some childhood experiences that gave rise to this fear.

Sarah's recovery journal

Excerpt 7

I believed I was 'good', but I had to be really careful not to be 'bold'. I tried to help everyone and be nice because otherwise someone would get annoyed and Mammy would start to cry and it would all turn horrible. I learned to be quiet, understanding and as kind as possible, because otherwise something would go wrong and they wouldn't like me, and I'd feel awful, and upset, and really lonely. I needed to feel loved and cared for, not neglected. But it seemed that their love was conditional. I had to work hard for their love and now I feel this with everyone.

I can't seem to ask for what I need. I'm afraid to and don't. The feeling of being afraid goes back a long way. I remember as a child coming downstairs from my bedroom, late at night, and standing for ages outside the kitchen door. I wanted a glass of water but I was terrified to go through the door and ask. I don't know why I found it so hard. I think I was terrified of being given out to and being told to get back to bed immediately, that it was too late for me to be up and that I had no business to be in the kitchen. In many different ways, I made efforts to ask for what I wanted but it often didn't get a favourable response. Many times over the course of my life, I remember saying to myself, 'I'll make an effort to say what I want but if it doesn't work, I'll never try again.' And at some point I simply gave up trying.

For Sarah, fear of upsetting others turned to a fear of asking for what she needed and the sense that even if she did ask, she would not be heard.

When you've lived for years believing that you have no right to ask for what you need, you stop listening to yourself and you gradually disown your needs. You may even decide that there is something wrong or shameful about asking for anything. Sarah learned that by ignoring her own needs and taking care of other people's, she could earn a place in their affections. While she was in hospital she was a 'model patient' who took care of many of the older people on the ward. The nurses regarded her kindness and helpfulness to others as evidence of a strong recovery but Sarah recognised herself how unhealthy such behaviour was.

Towards the end of her stay in hospital, Sarah began to change her pattern of relating to others. In the early part of her stay, she had communicated little of what she needed to the nursing staff and silently resented that they seemed so insensitive to what was going on for her. However, as she began to communicate more clearly what she needed, she was surprised to find just how supportive they were. She also learned to take care of her personal boundaries in a more appropriate way and not feel that she had to be completely open and compliant in relation to other people's requests. When a visiting relative asked some personal questions that Sarah found invasive, she calmly said she'd rather not talk about the issue. This was a significant shift for her and it made her feel uneasy and a little guilty. With time, however, she felt stronger and clearer about asking for what she needed and giving herself permission to protect her personal boundaries.

> ## Sarah's recovery journal
>
> ### *Excerpt 8*
>
> I now realise that when I spend all my time caring for and helping other patients, I'm actually isolating myself, disconnecting from myself, and devoting my time and attention to others rather than myself. I need to learn how to care for myself as well as other people. I need to listen to myself. I have to listen to my pain and not just that of other people. And I have to struggle with the pain inside me to try to release some of it bit by bit.

What can we learn from Sarah about relating to others?

- We each have a need to belong.
- Our childhood experiences teach each of us what to do to secure a sense of acceptance and belonging. Some of what we learn can end up hurting us as adults.
- Relationships are about give and take. My needs as well as those of others deserve to be respected.
- It is not wrong to be open with others about what you need. It helps them to know you better and creates the possibility of genuine friendship.

'I'm not good enough'

David had been very loved but overprotected all his life. He was bullied in school and, as a result, he felt that he wasn't as good as his peers. He feared any kind of competition that might expose his imagined 'incompetence'. His adolescence was marked by very happy memories of summer holidays, where he could 'play' without any pressure to compete and he enjoyed the easy company of friends. He also had very frightening memories of school, where he lived in fear of any kind of exam. He barely graduated school and took on a variety of third-level courses, all of which he left without completing. By his mid-twenties, he was unemployed, untrained and lacking any sense of direction about how he might secure a livelihood. Repeated failures to complete any course of training had gradually eroded all his self-confidence and resulted in severe depression.

Recovery for David involved building a positive self-image. He secured part-time employment and, within a year, had completed two of his unfinished courses and several other certificate courses. Each exam provoked tremendous fear and distress for him. He never believed he could pass and feared that the experience of yet another failure would be unbearably painful. He panicked in my office before each test and pleaded to be let off the hook. He tried to convince himself that each examination was unimportant and that he would be better off finding some other, less demanding, project. His lifelong protection against possible failure had been to run, but together we managed to enable him to accept his fear of failure and to confront it. His confidence grew with each success and carried him through the setbacks he also experienced. One year after his recovery, he dropped by to tell me he was off to the Far East to take up an exciting job opportunity. He commented on how he occasionally lapsed into self-criticism for all the years he had 'lost', but this never lasted too long.

I realise I wasted that time because I lacked self-confidence. I can do nothing about the past, but I can learn from it. I know how running away only reinforced my belief that I was incapable. I have learned how I need to act in ways that build up my self-confidence – by not running from challenges, by accepting there will be failures and setbacks. Rather than fear failure I now say to myself, 'If you're not failing, you're not learning.' And I've stopped looking for the instant fix. I accept that it takes time to build a sense of achievement.

David's self-image had been that he was essentially incompetent, and he had constructed a lifestyle where he had avoided situations that might expose this. Exams triggered this vulnerability in him and caused him to feel anxious and depressed. His recovery required a lot of courage because he had to let go of his key survival strategy – 'Avoid failure at all costs because it will be unbearable.' By confronting his greatest fear – that he was incompetent – he discovered he was both intelligent and courageous.

What can we learn from David's recovery?

- Your self-image is shaped by key experiences in your life.
- Your self-image is the story you tell yourself about what kind of person you are.
- Sometimes, the 'story' holds you back.
- When you run from what you fear, your fear becomes stronger.
- Facing your fears takes courage, but conquering them feels wonderful.

I'm ashamed of who I am

The insecurities you have about yourself never go away completely. What changes in recovery is your ability to understand where these insecurities have come from and to not be drawn into believing they represent the 'truth'. You also learn to identify the kinds of situations that provoke these insecurities and what you can do to support yourself when your confidence is shaken. As you recover, you gradually discover that while your insecurities are part of who you are, they are not the whole story.

Your true identity is large enough and strong enough for you to accept and even befriend these insecurities.

Alan was a successful professional man in his late thirties. His childhood was marked by abuse and obscenity on the part of his mother. She would regularly dress him in girls' underwear and later when he was at play with his friends, she would pull down his pants and humiliate him while they looked on. He was constantly told he was 'bad', and was sent to school with a sense that it was a waste of time because he was 'stupid'.

He worked hard to prove his mother wrong. But throughout his life, he was riddled with shame and self-doubt. He repeatedly had thoughts of being 'bad' and despite his considerable achievements, he felt he had achieved very little in life compared to his friends. His shame triggered several episodes of depression in his adult life, and it took him a long time to ask for help.

Therapy gradually helped him to recover a sense of his basic goodness and resilience. He moved from seeing himself as something shameful to seeing in himself a young boy who had survived unbelievable abuse and who had still managed to grow into an adult capable of loving others.

One day, he arrived to our session having done something that expressed his appreciation to that young boy. He had decided to do this because he wanted to finally make peace with his childhood and let go the shame he had felt all of his life.

His journey from home to school each morning had been especially difficult for him. He would leave home having endured a tirade of abuse, with his homework incomplete, and terrified of what further criticisms he might receive during the day. As an adult who was recovering from depression, he realised that the little boy was still part of him and that he needed encouragement and support. So one morning, he returned to the house that had been his family home at the precise time that he would have left for school. He remembered what standing there had felt like when he was eight years old. And then he walked the journey from home to school imagining himself in the company of this little boy.

As he walked he spoke to this little boy. He told him how proud he was of him and how unfair it was that he was sent out into life so unprepared and unsupported by his parents. He told him how proud he was of the way he had kept going and not given up when things were so dark. He promised he would always be there for him from now on.

Our self-image comes down to the way in which we view ourselves. We can view ourselves as flawed victims or as 'heroes' who survived many experiences that hurt and confused us. Our self-image also depends on the way we 'talk' to ourselves. It's so easy to speak to ourselves with contempt when we get something wrong; but we will never experience recovery until we find in ourselves an attitude that is best described as kindness. Recovery shifts gear when you begin to look at yourself with appreciation and when you start accepting the person you are. Kindness and patience make an enormous difference to the way you feel inside your own skin.

There is a poem that captures the importance of kindness better than any words I can find.

Kindness
By Naomi Shihab Nye

Before you know what kindness really is
you must lose things,
feel the future dissolve in a moment
like salt in a weakened broth.
What you held in your hand,
what you counted and carefully saved,
all this must go so you know
how desolate the landscape can be

between the regions of kindness.
How you ride and ride
thinking the bus will never stop,
the passengers eating maize and chicken
will stare out the window forever.

Before you learn the tender gravity of kindness,
you must travel where the Indian in a white poncho
lies dead by the side of the road.
You must see how this could be you,
how he too was someone
who journeyed through the night
with plans and the simple breath
that kept him alive.

Before you know kindness
as the deepest thing inside,
you must know sorrow
as the other deepest thing.
You must wake up with sorrow.
You must speak to it till your voice
catches the thread of all sorrows
and you see the size of the cloth.
Then it is only kindness
that makes sense anymore,
only kindness that ties your shoes
and sends you out into the day
to mail letters and purchase bread,
only kindness that raises its head
from the crowd of the world to say
it is I you have been looking for,
and then goes with you every where
like a shadow or a friend.

Summary

In order to recover, we need to see the harm that we have been doing by continuing to hold on to the negative image of ourselves that we formed in our childhoods. We need to see that as long as we cut other people out of our life, we will remain isolated. To be ourselves with others is the goal of our recovery. This frees us from needless pressure and frustration, and it opens up our life to possibilities of lasting friendship and intimacy. To be yourself is as much a gift we receive from others, as it is a choice that we make. Success depends on finding people we can trust, people who see us for who we really are and with whom we feel safe enough to be our true selves.

Self-help exercise

Consider the following questions and give yourself time to answer them.

- What were some of the important messages you picked up from your family about how to survive in this world?
- In what ways have these messages helped you – how have they helped you to become *strong*? In what ways have they set you up for certain kinds of problems – how have you become *vulnerable* as a result of these messages?
- What do you need to change to help you accept your vulnerabilities and not get carried away by them?
- What could you say to yourself that would allow you to be kinder to yourself when things don't work out the way you hoped and planned?

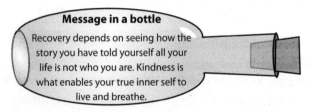

Message in a bottle

Recovery depends on seeing how the story you have told yourself all your life is not who you are. Kindness is what enables your true inner self to live and breathe.

CHAPTER 6

Putting it all together: Tom's story

One Sunday, an hour after returning from coaching the junior football team, Tom had his 'heart attack'. His GP was summoned and, finding Tom collapsed on the dining room floor with an alarmingly low pulse, dispatched him by ambulance to the local Accident and Emergency. Relatives were contacted 'just in case' and gathered around the cardiac monitor. Their respectful silence and concerned faces spoke volumes. Tom got the message: he was 43, happily married with five children and had a good job, but his number was up. How would they cope after he was gone?

Surprisingly, it was of no comfort to Tom when the suspected 'heart attack' was ruled out and when his doctors decided his problem was something much less sinister, Acute Pericarditis, an inflammation of the tissue around the heart. In five days, he was treated and discharged from hospital with the all clear from the medical staff. But instead of feeling relieved he became depressed, and his depression continued for the next six years. Two 10-week psychiatric admissions, ECT and drug treatment did little to help. When he eventually was referred for cognitive therapy, those years of relentless misery had taken their toll. He didn't feel much like talking.

Tom was slight in stature and naturally shy. He sat in my office and seemed unsure of why he was there. I was yet another in a long series of professionals he'd encountered. By his demeanour, it was clear that he didn't believe I could do any more for him than others before me. The referral note from his doctor described him as a man with a negative attitude to most things in his life. He had a six-year history of depression but treatment had not helped to shift his pessimism.

Tom worked hard for his family and he expected little in return other than that his children would leave the family home with a self-confidence that he'd always lacked. He described his own father as a particularly harsh man who 'broke his spirit' as a young boy. When Tom reached adolescence, he dropped out of school, left his home and started work. By 19, he was a successful bread salesman and a series of promotions followed, he got married and set up a home. He now worked as a salesman for a very successful company and he was a much-valued employee. His loyalty to the company was uncompromising and he worked over and above the call of duty. He had five children who adored him as much as he did them. So why had he turned away from life and lapsed into such an immovable depression?

I didn't want to live. I just wasn't able to face living. I thought everybody could see me as I felt and what I felt in my mind was so horrifying. I couldn't bear to think that people could see me in that way. I withdrew from everything I was used to. I had no confidence in going to meet customers or to collect the debts the company was owed. I'd find myself driving up the road and having to stop and come home. I basically just wanted to sit in a room by myself and be left alone.

For six years, he shut himself off from the world and sank deeper and deeper into misery. He remained at work but came home every evening and fell asleep in the chair after dinner. He showed no interest in activities that had been previously a source of pleasure for him, like gardening, football, being with his children and meeting friends. The family watched his decline and wondered whether they were perhaps the cause of his pain. They walked on eggshells around him, making few demands on him and trying not to discommode him. As time passed, they relied less and less on him to participate in normal family life. They stopped expecting him to be 'Dad'.

> I felt myself retreating away from the wife and children because of the fear that there was something there that they could see – 'Daddy is going mad.' They weren't saying anything like this but I felt in my mind they were saying it.

Because of his depression, Tom was convinced that he was worthless, incompetent and unlovable. It was an enormous effort for him just to get through each day. The most painful part of it all was that his torment seemed to be endless. Not surprisingly, he began to consider whether the only way out of his pain might be death.

> I did feel that it would be the best thing for everybody if I ran the car over a cliff or ended my life in some way. But something inside me said, 'Don't be stupid', and thank God that something stopped me.

Even when he was surrounded by his wife and children, Tom felt utterly alone. He felt that this was probably something that every person who was depressed experienced because it's so hard for friends and loved ones to grasp what it feels like to be depressed.

> People don't understand depression. If you have a broken arm, everybody has all the pity in the world for you. If you

have a broken leg, people will help you up a stairs, open a door for you. But if you have depression, nobody knows only yourself, so you are living with it yourself. They say cancer is a killer, but depression is the worst disease out. It's a prison sentence that seems to go on for ever.

His first professional contact was with his GP, who diagnosed depression and suggested a referral to a psychiatrist for medication. At one point, he was on six to eight tablets daily, but, as can happen in some cases, they did little to help him. Hospital admission was arranged on two different occasions.

Hospitalisation didn't help me in the condition I was in. I felt I was just a number. Don't get me wrong. I know the country is full of patients. I didn't want any special kind of treatment, but what I would have loved was for somebody to come and sit beside the bed and talk to me about how I was, and what my problem was. To explain it to me. To be given tablets and left there by yourself, your meals served up, and staff dropping in to say hello and goodbye, wasn't enough for me. I wanted to know what was happening, why I felt the way I did and what the end product was going to be.

When he was hospitalised, Tom's depression was viewed as primarily a medical problem. He was considered to have a chemical imbalance that could only be corrected with medication. While this helped to ease the pain he experienced, it didn't address the underlying causes of his depression. Electroconvulsive therapy (ECT) was also administered during his hospital admission. This is a treatment that delivers a very mild electric shock to the brain and thereby alters the brain chemistry. For some people with severe chronic depression, ECT has been found to have dramatic benefits in lifting their mood, even if only for a short time. However, this treatment did little to improve Tom's situation. What he had kept asking for was someone to talk to and, finally, after six years, he was referred for cognitive therapy.

This therapy is based on a very simple truth that how we react to events in our life all depends on how we think about these events. For example, if you are walking down the street and see an old friend on the opposite side of the street walk right by without acknowledging you are there, you could react in a number of different ways. If you decided that your friend must not have seen you, you might feel briefly disappointed but very quickly forget it ever happened. But if you saw them pass right by you and thought, 'Why is he ignoring me? I must have done something to really upset him. I am so stupid, I just can't seem to keep friends', then it would be very natural to feel deeply upset by this experience and probably feel down for several hours afterwards.

Tom's depression was triggered by the physical health crisis he experienced, but no one had ever explored what this experience had meant to him, how he had interpreted it at the time. This was the key to understanding why he had become *so* upset and why he had sunk into a deep depression in the years that followed it.

Together, we revisited the day he had his 'heart attack' and we went back over each moment of his ordeal. We discovered that what had troubled him the most was not actually his imagined 'cardiac arrest', or the threat of death, or the potential loss of his family, but rather a deep insecurity that had been reactivated on that day; an old wound from his childhood that had been reopened and that had remained open since.

As he lay on the dining room floor waiting for the ambulance to arrive, he heard his father's voice saying clearly, 'You're a loser, you can never be counted on, you just don't have what it takes to make it.' Tom interpreted this crisis as proof that his dad was right; that he was unreliable and that his family should never count on him to provide for them. He interpreted his physical crisis as proof that what he had always feared most about himself was true. To protect the people he loved most in the world, he deliberately started to put a distance between himself and his family. Eventually, they stopped counting on him, and Tom interpreted this as further proof that he had little to offer them. The following diagram illustrates the sequence of events that triggered Tom's depression and the vicious cycle of negative thinking and self-defeating behaviour that kept it alive for six years.

TOM'S DEPRESSION

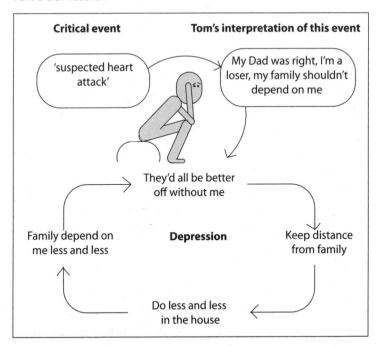

In our sessions together, Tom began to see how the negative view of himself that he'd carried since childhood was at the root of his depression.

> I was made feel very inferior as I was growing up … that I was never good enough for anything or to be anything. When the 'heart attack' came, it was like 'proof' that everything I had heard was true.

He recalled a critical event that had sparked the poor relationship he'd had with his father. When he was eight years old, his sister, who was aged 12, died. In a family of 11 siblings, he had never been that close to his mother, and this particular sister had been the person who had mothered him. On the morning she died, his father had come into his bedroom and told him he wouldn't be going to school that day. He watched her funeral pass by through his front window and felt completely bewildered by it all. Nothing was ever the same afterwards and his relationship with his father deteriorated badly.

> It basically had to do with my dad. But then I didn't blame him either. The more I looked at things, the more I realised it basically wasn't his fault. I lost a sister who was like a mother to me. My dad also lost a daughter whom he thought the world of. And I feel he looked upon me as though I should have died and my sister should have lived. So he downed me always, no matter what I did. He never thought me capable of any good. I didn't dislike him; I loved him. I did everything possible to please him, but it didn't make any difference to him. He just didn't seem to relate to me at all. It was a pity really because it would have been a better life for both of us if he had realised my feelings for him. He was depressed when he lost my sister but I lost as much as he lost.

Deep down, Tom had always believed his dad was disappointed in him and that he had good reason to be, and so Tom overworked all his life to compensate for this imagined deficiency. His coping was by any standard impressive, but when he was incapacitated that Sunday afternoon, he had relived, with complete conviction, the shameful self-image he had formed as a boy.

Tom continued to live out this negative belief in the six years that followed. He adopted a passive and ineffectual role at home because he believed it was in his family's best interest that they should not depend on him. In his mind, this was the best he could do to avoid letting them down, which would have been more than he could bear, and which he believed would hurt them too. For the first time, he understood why he was behaving as he was in respect to those he loved most in the world.

As he recalled these formative childhood experiences, the intense pain of a young eight-year-old boy, whose sister had died tragically and whose father seemed to turn against him viciously in the years that followed, became very vivid. Despair slowly gave way to anger as he struggled against that negative inner voice he had internalised, which continued to drain his energy and his will to live.

Tom's early attempts to talk back to what he called his mental 'bully' with the evidence of a life lived out steadily, faithfully and successfully were timid at best. After a number of therapy sessions, he visited his sister's grave with the intention of telling her for the first time how upset he had been. However, he was unable to do this. His explanation on returning to therapy was that his father was buried next to her and he could imagine his father criticising him for being so weak.

With time, he became stronger and challenged the things his father had said to him in anger. As he remembered the pain of his past, he also recognised the strength of the bullied child within him, the child that had survived, grown into an adult and had given a good life to others. He recognised too that his dad's behaviour was an expression of the pain he struggled with, rather than anything that he, Tom, had provoked or deserved.

To prove his dad wrong, Tom had always pushed himself hard and believed that if he ever did let down his own children, his father would win. What drove him was his belief that, 'If I do not provide completely for my children, then I will prove myself to be an incompetent loser.' Living rigidly by this rule left him worried constantly that something might happen to threaten his job. As a result, he worked seven days a week, hoping to establish himself as indispensable, but actually increased the risks to his health and putting his job and his life in serious jeopardy.

While it was an immense relief for Tom to understand the root cause of his depression, the real challenge for him in his recovery was to expose the lie that he was 'unreliable'. To break the grip of his negative thinking, he started to act differently around his family, taking time to re-establish a relationship with each of them and supporting each of them in whatever way he could. As his belief in himself returned, he noticed when his negative thinking became active in his mind, and he was able to see these thoughts for what they were, rather than assume they were true. Eventually, he was able to address the root of his problems – his relationship with his dad – and to stop running from him.

I did everything. I went to the graveyard. I discussed with him what he had wanted of me. As sure as hell if there is a heaven we're going to have a hell of a chat. I got it out into the open and had a good look at it and I saw that my negative thinking was a ghost of despair and depression. It was a voice telling me something that was completely untrue about myself. I learned to accept it was untrue and the more I did, the more courage I got to fight it. Basically, I was able to fight with him to let go of me, that I didn't deserve what he did and what he was still doing in my head. That I wasn't the type of person that he thought I was; that I was going to succeed and that he wasn't going to stop me. It was a hard struggle, because he had a terrible grip on me. If you love someone, they have a grip on you. And I did love my dad. And I'd tell him that tomorrow if I met him because I still love him. But I didn't deserve what he was doing to me, because I wasn't the type of person that he had made me out to be.

As Tom began to believe that he could be counted on, his relationship with his family changed. He began to take more responsibility at home and gradually he became 'Dad' again. It was hard at first for the family to adjust to his behaviour change because they were so used to seeing him as a quite passive, self-centred figure. Meetings were arranged between him and his wife to discuss how he could re-enter the family, and to talk about her difficulty in trusting that his improvement would last. Her support was critical in enabling Tom to return to being a father and a husband.

As he reworked his relationships at home, Tom also related differently to others outside the home. He took more initiative with colleagues at work and with friends he'd been neglecting. His self-confidence steadily returned and his depression lifted.

I'm better able to face things now. I'm not afraid to express how I feel to others. Before I sat back and was silent even if I didn't agree with what was being said. I would have thought that anything I had to say was stupid. Now I believe in myself and I say what I think.

As Tom's therapy drew to a close, we considered the possible situations that might cause him to relapse. We discussed some practical coping skills that would carry him beyond therapy and help him for the rest of his life. In the five years that have passed since his therapy ended, Tom has been in touch on occasions. He has never since experienced the despair he endured for those six bleak years of his life. He has had bad days, some very difficult life experiences, but he has coped with them without letting himself be drawn back into chronic depression.

> My routine to survive is that I go out each morning and I say to myself, 'Today is going to be better than yesterday.' No matter what problem I meet, I say, 'It's only a problem, I will deal with it.' If I think it's too much for me, I walk away from it and I come back to it with fresh thoughts the next day. Before it would get me down and I wouldn't sleep at night. Now I see each problem as just another part of life, and tomorrow it will be better. I'm coping, I'm living, I enjoy what I want to enjoy. And I am quite happy with what I have. That's it.

As therapy draws to a close people become clearer about the elements of their life experience that have contributed to their depression and, at the same time, they begin to see these experiences in a new way. Although the painful elements of their stories remain the same, the meaning changes. Painful memories can now be accepted and they feel compassion for people who may have been hurt in similar ways. Tom also realised that his father's abusive behaviour had given him a vital insight in raising his own children.

> My dad really taught me how important it is to build up a person's feeling of self-confidence. The human spirit can be easily broken … At least my children can never say I did that

to them and that's the most important thing I've ever given them. My dad gave me that. Maybe it's OK I went through what he put me through to teach me that, but maybe it's OK to stop doing that to myself now.

CHAPTER 7

Supporting a person who is depressed

L iving with someone who is depressed can be very challenging for families and friends. Loved ones can feel as confused as the sufferer and become worn out, feel guilty and be exasperated by their inability to help. In this chapter there are some suggestions to help you genuinely support the sufferer, while not being drawn into the darkness of their depression.

For convenience, we can think in terms of two different stages in living with this problem: the stage where neither you nor the sufferer knows what's wrong and their mood and their behaviour become steadily worse, and a further stage when everyone accepts that there is a problem which may require some form of help.

Living with someone who has not yet accepted they have a problem

In the early stages of depression, a person may deny there is anything wrong and gradually cut themselves off from you and everyone else. You try everything to lift their spirits but nothing works. In moments of serious exasperation, you resort to telling them to 'cheer up' and 'snap out of it'. This only aggravates the situation even more. Confusion sets in and you come up with all kinds of explanations for what might be happening: 'Is there something wrong physically with them?', 'Is it our relationship?',

'Is it me?', 'Should we be living somewhere else?' You struggle alone with these questions, because it is not easy to talk about your concerns with somebody who is withdrawn and non-communicative. Eventually, your explanations may come down to blaming them for being 'selfish' or blaming yourself for being 'inadequate'.

The pitfalls at this stage are *isolation* and *confusion*. The isolation into which the person who is depressed sinks can exert a gravitational pull on everyone around them. Almost without realising it, the family can become cut off from their normal social supports. Because the sufferer does not find it easy to have visitors, friends and relatives are no longer invited to drop in. Children don't invite their friends in, and neighbours don't drop by casually, as they can sense a change in the atmosphere.

To survive this stage, it is important that you let someone you trust know what's happening. Someone who can help you to see that you are not imagining the pressures you are under and that what's happening is impacting on everyone concerned.

Talking about it with the right person helps you to get some perspective on the situation and to see what might be helpful. This, in turn, makes it easier to talk to the person who is depressed without blaming anybody and with a clear intention of figuring out what might help everyone deal with the situation more effectively.

The person who is depressed may have no idea how much of an impact their mood is having on those around them. You may need to tell them what is happening to you at an emotional level. Be very simple and specific about how you feel. And, as far as possible, speak slowly and calmly. People who are sinking into depression find it impossible to cope with intense emotion or even the slightest criticism. Try to share your own feelings, rather than blame them for what they are doing 'wrong'.

For example, saying:

> When you sit in silence at the dinner table, I feel lonely and cut off and start asking myself all kinds of questions about what I might have done wrong to upset you.

may be a lot easier for them to hear than if you say:

> Why are you doing this to all of us? Why are you being so selfish?

If the person's state of mind continues to worsen and they seem unable to acknowledge that they have a problem, it may be important for you to seek professional advice on how best to respond and be helpful. You could consult with your GP or some local counsellor, and discuss the problems that you are experiencing being around the person who is depressed. You are not blaming them, you are not seeking to betray loyalties, you are simply trying to access the support *you* need to stay grounded and to look after yourself, your family and the needs of any children who may be involved. At the end of this book, there are some addresses of websites and helplines that may be relevant.

What one woman found hardest in this phase of her husband's depression was that she had to 'detach to survive'. In her mind, this seemed so 'selfish' because sometimes the best she could do was to walk out of the room and leave him in his despair. She had to challenge one of her beliefs she had been raised with: 'If you really love someone, you suffer along with them no matter what it takes.' She had three children and, over time, she learned that she couldn't make her husband better and that 'to try means you end up sinking into depression yourself, and being no good to anybody'.

If the problem reaches a crisis point and a person seems unable or unwilling to accept that they need help, it may be necessary for you to step back until they do accept their problems. This might even involve leaving them for a period of time. You would not do this lightly, but when you no longer see any other way of communicating to them how painful the situation has become for everyone, this may be the only way to reach them. You may still maintain phone communication and reassure them of your support. Your intention is not to abandon or hurt them, but to encourage them to overcome their denial and face their problems.

One of the fears that loved ones experience is that if they do not do exactly what the person who is depressed wants, they run the risk of losing them through suicide. If it's a young person who is in the grip of depression, walking out may simply not be an option. I receive countless calls from parents who feel helpless in situations like this and who are completely at a loss about what they should do. On the one hand, they want to be tough and insist that their son or daughter do something to help themselves; on the other hand, they are afraid that if they take their eyes off them for even a moment, something really bad could happen.

What I say to parents in a crisis like this is, first of all, to trust that the fact that their concern about their son's or daughter's welfare really does matter to that young person. And while they will not be thanked for it at the time, their steady presence and their willingness to 'hang in' with them is deeply important and appreciated. I'm not saying they will never hear words of thanks – it is very likely they will – but such words may take time.

The second point that I make to parents is that they should consider whether there is someone in this young person's life whom they might trust. Perhaps there is an uncle, aunt, teacher or youth leader who knows this young person and cares about them. It is often easier to open up to an adult who is not a parent and with whom we don't have an emotionally complex relationship. For one thing, the young person may be terrified to open up to their parents because they fear that what they say will be very upsetting for the parent to hear. Someone close to the young person, but outside the immediate family circle, may provide a less complicated option from the young person's point of view.

There are also a number of ways that a parent can help their son or daughter indirectly. I often recommend that they consider seeing someone professional themselves, whether the young person agrees to come along or not. It is all the better of course if both parents and the young person can sit down together as a family with a therapist and hear from each other what each of them needs. But if communication is at an all time low, then a 'family meeting' may not be an option.

What's important is that the parent(s) acknowledge that this is a really hard situation for themselves and that *they* may need help just as much as the young person. It's often interesting what emerges when parents consult with a therapist for themselves. They may discover that they each have their own particular difficulty with their young person's experience and yet they have never really communicated this to each other. Their lack of communication can give rise to any number of tensions in the young person who may be getting mixed messages from them. A consultation can offer the opportunity to resolve the tensions that result from very different points of view on what's causing their child's pain. When the air is clear between parents, it is much easier for them to think about what might work with their child and then for them to take a consistent and united approach in their interactions with the young person.

Finally, there is the situation where the young person's life may be seriously at risk. In situations like this, it can be hard to know where to turn or who to talk to. Services for young people (aged 12–25) are thin on the ground. What you need in this situation is someone who can direct you to a service that will appreciate that while the young person's life may be at risk, they are unlikely to take the first step in attending a service by themselves. Your GP can identify the most appropriate local health service and request someone there to make a home visit. A letter from the parent(s) themselves to the clinical director of the local health service can also be an effective way to communicate a sense of urgency.

Living with someone who accepts they are depressed

When a person you love accepts that they need to talk to someone about their depression, life gets a little easier. Tensions within your relationship and your family ease slightly, if not considerably. This is a critical first step but there are many challenges ahead to be faced. The following suggestions may help you to navigate this phase of their recovery.

Dealing with cruel outbursts

People who feel badly about themselves frequently take it out on people they love. They become exhausted with carrying a sense of 'badness' inside and project some of their bad feelings onto those around them. Perhaps it is because these are the only people they feel they can trust; perhaps because they do not want anyone outside their immediate family to see the dark side of their problems.

Accusations are hurled at loved ones blaming them for everything that is wrong: 'It's all your fault, you never support me', 'You never really respected me and you've always treated me as if I'm stupid.'

The most hurtful comments are often those directed at

children. One man who was known for his gentleness and sensitivity to others was given to making cruel comments to his children when he was depressed. He would tell them that he regretted ever having them and he would repeatedly threaten to get rid of them. When he recovered he recalled these comments and bitterly regretted them. His relationship with his children suffered badly, and it took many years to repair. His openness and honest apology to them when he had recovered was crucial in rebuilding this relationship. From the children's perspective, they mentioned years later that what helped them to overcome the hurt their father had inflicted was being able to separate who he was as a person from his depression.

The cruel things that a person who is depressed may say are spoken from a place of deep self-hate. To want to react in anger is perfectly understandable, but more often this aggravates the situation. There is a point where you simply may need to leave the room, but if you can speak to the hurt and fear in a person that lies behind these destructive comments, you may find that their tone softens.

Thus, an unhelpful response to unreasonable accusations may be something like:

That's so unfair, I've always been here for you.

While this may seem completely justified, it only fuels the fire of self-hate and anger that grips the sufferer in that moment. A more effective response might be one that acknowledges the confusion and pain behind their tirade:

It sounds as if you're feeling bad about everything including our relationship, as if there is nothing good in the world to hold on to.

Remaining calm in the face of another's distress

When you are feeling happy and clear-headed, the complaints of a person who is depressed seem completely unreasonable. Why would they have such a poor opinion of themselves? Don't they appreciate all they have achieved? Don't they realise how much people care about them?

The temptation is naturally to encourage them to think 'positively'. But someone who is experiencing depression cannot make this shift easily and they can feel even more 'stupid' for not being able to 'think positively'. There is a time to challenge negative thinking, but there is a time to respect that someone is severely upset and needs companionship rather than logic. Sometimes that person needs to vent, and the best you can do is to let them vent and not take any of it personally. It's not up to you to make them see their lives as the gift you know it to be. What you need to do is to steady yourself, take a few breaths and let what they are saying flow in one ear and out the other. Take the pressure off yourself to cheer them up. Trust that your calm presence is what they need most. Your job is to look after yourself rather than to fix them.

Some human suffering must simply be lived. Attempts to relieve another's suffering can be a subtle refusal to accept and respect their experience. Some black moods have to be endured for some hours or days before they begin to heal. When the break comes, dialogue becomes easier and there may well be a place for helping loved ones remember positive aspects of their life that have become eclipsed in depression.

Give space but don't isolate

For parents with young adult children going through depression, there is often a conflict about how much space to offer and how much they should check in on how their child is doing. There is a delicate balance to be achieved between giving someone a respectful amount of space and isolating them through complete neglect. You have to walk a difficult path between, on the one hand, suffocating them and, on the other, abandoning them.

Having a regular routine where you can check in briefly with a young person may be enough to keep in touch rather than making constant enquiries about how they are doing. Such an occasion should be a time and place where you both feel relaxed. It may be when you're both driving home, or following a meal when everyone has finished up and left. Find a moment in the week that works for you as much as for them, don't probe too deeply; just ask some simple questions that you know they can answer. Acknowledge whatever is tough for them and respect them for continuing to hang in there.

Believe in their ability to get through this

The most important message you can convey to someone struggling with depression is your faith in his or her ability to fight it and to come through it. Maybe they require some professional help, but ultimately recovery will be something they achieve when they find their inner strength. It will be their choice, and their victory, and they need to sense from you that you believe they can do it.

Keep your own family and social life going

Don't allow another person's depression to drain your energy and completely disrupt your personal life. Keep in touch with your own work projects, leisure pursuits, and especially with friends who nurture and support you. Don't let go of whatever sustains you. There will be times when you will need to say to a loved one, 'I need to leave now and give myself a break.' This may seem harsh, if they are in a difficult space, but you need time for yourself in order to be able to be there for them and the rest of the family when you return.

Don't underestimate children who may be involved

Children have an uncanny way of picking up atmospheres and tensions within the home. Their apparent silence and indifference to what is happening should never be taken as a sign that they are unaffected by the suffering of a parent who is depressed.

It may be appropriate in the early stages to try to protect them from the suffering of a parent, but to continue to deny something is wrong, when they clearly sense this to be the case, only serves to confuse and worry them more. Children can generally cope very well with knowing someone else is unwell or upset, but they do not do at all well with feeling that they are inflicting or causing that upset for a parent. At some point, it is best to be very honest about the fact that the sufferer is upset and feeling bad about themselves. This locates the problem where it belongs and protects children, who are inclined to blame themselves for whatever they sense is wrong in the home.

It is not uncommon for people in depression to say very cruel things to children when they are in a dark mood and these types of comments need to be addressed rather than be allowed to fester in the mind of the child. I remember seeing the family of a man who had been depressed for many years but who refused to seek help. His wife and three of his four children attended for an initial session and I remarked on the absence of the daughter who was 14 at that time . They explained that this would be much too upsetting for her and they had arranged to meet me without her knowledge. I had not met this child but in principle I found this to be an uncomfortable arrangement, so I requested that she might be brought along to the next meeting. At all subsequent meetings, she turned out to be the person who most accurately portrayed the atmosphere of the home and who could relate most sensitively to her father in his different moods. Her insights guided me in helping her family. It was also apparent that this young girl was trying desperately hard to make everyone else happy, while she herself struggled with problems of sleepwalking, bed-wetting and an inability to concentrate at school. By allowing her to be present and voice her concerns, I was able to communicate to her that we would look after her dad and free her of that sole responsibility.

Summary

It can be hard to know how best to support a loved one when they are in the grips of depression. On the one hand, it's easy to be intolerant and critical; while on the other hand there is the danger of becoming drawn into their experience and becoming exhausted. Find someone to support you and keep you grounded. Attend to your work and do whatever is nurturing for you. Cruel things said in the midst of rage and despair may cause deep wounds that linger long after the depression has lifted. Know how much you can tolerate and recognise when you've reached your limit. There is only so much you can do. To try to do more will wear you down to the point where you have nothing to give. Taking care of yourself enables you to be present to another's pain without being consumed by it. Your presence and belief in them enables them to calm down and find hope.

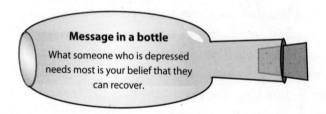

Message in a bottle
What someone who is depressed needs most is your belief that they can recover.

PART THREE

Living with Yourself

CHAPTER 8

How 'mindfulness' can support recovery

Recovery from depression is a journey rather than a destination. It begins when we refuse to believe that being depressed is the best we can hope for. It takes time, and there are lots of ups and downs. It is a path we walk where we slowly rediscover that there is something good inside us that we can trust; an inner strength that cannot be broken. Through recovery, we learn to rest in our own skin, to listen to and to take care of the person we are.

But the experience of depression can leave us feeling very unsure of *who we are*. Even on a good day, when we feel happy in ourselves, there may be a fear in the back of our minds that depression will come back, that it will creep up on us out of nowhere and take over our lives again before we know what is happening.

To cope with our fear of depression, we develop unhelpful habits. We speed from one event to another, from one experience to the next, without giving ourselves time to appreciate and savour small, everyday miracles. We seldom take time to stop and check in with ourselves, to simply be with ourselves, to rest. When we are troubled, we do not know how to look after ourselves. When we notice our mood dropping, we say to ourselves 'This shouldn't be happening' or 'For heaven's sake surely you're not still letting something like X get to you' or 'Just forget about it, watch some TV, you'll be OK tomorrow'.

When we feel upset, we want to run from ourselves, to push away our distress or to 'fix' it as quickly as possible. While these reactions might be widely used coping mechanisms, they seldom work for people vulnerable to depression. In fact, we now know that *suppression* (pushing away painful feelings) and *rumination* (fighting with ourselves for feeling the way we do) can provoke a relapse into depression.

Depression can recur with alarming frequency once a person has had two or more episodes. Finding a way to reduce relapse turns out to be the single greatest challenge for people who have experienced depression. Long-term medication protects many people from relapse, but the problem is that when the medication is discontinued, the majority of these people become depressed quickly. So while their medication may be protective, it is not curative. The support of a relationship with a skilful psychotherapist on a long-term basis is also an option that works, but this is not easily available and for many people it can be an overly expensive option.

The challenge to find some alternative sustainable way of preventing relapse really challenged researchers in the last decade of the 20th century. What they discovered was that a structured, eight-week training course in *mindfulness* reduced relapse in recurrent major depression by 50 per cent. These studies have shown that relapse is not inevitable. Mindfulness is now taught all over the world to groups of people in hospitals, in clinics and in local communities.

Mindfulness means resting in the present moment, with full awareness. When we are mindful, we bring our attention back to whatever is happening in our lives. We notice the good things that are happening in our lives, and we enjoy moments in a day that could easily pass us by: the smile on a child's face, the sensation of the breeze against our skin, the way sunlight plays on the water, the patterns windscreen wipers make on a rainy day. When we practise mindfulness on a daily basis, we also become more finely tuned to our inner lives. We learn to notice and to accept difficulties as they emerge, rather than trying to push them away and suppress them. We learn to steady ourselves in the face of strong emotions, and to disengage from negative thought patterns (rumination) before they gather steam and gain the upper hand.

Mindfulness gives us a gentle way to respond to distress. Rather than 'reacting' to our distress, it encourages us to 'relate' to it. Rather than pushing difficult feelings away, it enables us to 'hold' them in our awareness and to see what they may be trying to tell us about our lives. When we learn how to be with our experience without being overwhelmed by it, we can respond creatively rather than in a frightened, defensive manner.

Often, the most effective method of dealing with our painful moods is to gently acknowledge what's happening and let them be, without being pulled into doing battle with them.

These next few chapters will show you how to practise mindfulness and will enable you to experience the powerful way it can support your recovery from depression. There are many excellent writers on this subject – many of whom I have included in the list of references and resources at the back of this book – but, in my own professional life, I have benefited from three teachers in particular: Thich Nhat Hanh, Jon Kabat-Zinn and Mark Williams. These people have been pioneers in bringing the practice of mindfulness into healthcare. And at different stages of my own personal and professional development, they have been my teachers.

Much of what is taught today on mindfulness courses has its origin in the writings of Thich Nhat Hanh, a Zen monk who is also a poet and a peace activist who was nominated for the Nobel Peace Prize by Martin Luther King.

In the Vietnam War, Thich Nhat Hanh (who prefers to be called 'Thay', the Vietnam word for teacher) established a movement to try to bring peace between North and South Vietnam. Many of his family and close friends were murdered in the course of this work for peace. He was heartbroken and he became so depressed in the early 1960s that he was hospitalised.

His depression was severe and unresponsive to any kind of intervention and his doctors reached a point where they considered the only option left to them was electroconvulsive therapy (ECT). Thay chose not to accept this option. Instead, he gradually worked his way out of depression, with support from those around him and particularly by practising mindfulness. He has always credited mindfulness with saving his life. In 1972, he wrote about the importance of mindfulness to him in his recovery in a book entitled *The Miracle of Mindfulness*. Since that time, he has published more than 100 books on the practice.

Thay was exiled from Vietnam because of his peace work and he took refuge in the United States. He began to give retreats across America in the 1970s. In 1979, a young man called Jon Kabat-Zinn was present at one of these retreats. As he listened, Jon realised how relevant Thay's teachings on mindfulness were for the people he had been treating at that time, for chronic medical conditions in a general hospital at the University of Massachusetts in Boston.

Jon began to incorporate Thay's teachings with people who suffered with chronic pain and stress. He adapted Thay's teaching on mindfulness into a structured eight-week course, which he called 'mindfulness-based stress reduction' (MBSR). In the mid-1990s, Jon's work came to the attention of three leading cognitive therapy researchers in the field of depression, Zindel Segal, John

Teasdale and Mark Williams. These researchers had become aware of how serious the problem of relapse was for people who had experienced depression. In mindfulness training, they saw a possible way for people to protect themselves from repeated relapses. In the mid-1990s, they visited Jon Kabat-Zinn to learn more about this method.

As they attended Jon's course, and watched the way he worked with people who were experiencing pain and distress, they saw how mindfulness could also be helpful to people who lived with the fear of becoming depressed. They returned to the UK and began to apply mindfulness with groups of people who had experienced many episodes of depression. They published the results of their work in 2002, in a ground-breaking book entitled *Mindfulness-Based Cognitive Therapy.*

This book describes in detail how the authors adapted mindfulness to work with depression. Their research has been replicated with consistently positive results (each study showing a reduction in rate of relapse by at least 50 per cent) and this work has given rise to an explosion of mindfulness courses in hospitals and clinics right across the world of mental health. Mindfulness has since been shown to benefit not only people vulnerable to depression, but also people with different kinds of health and mental health problems.

My own writing draws on all the above sources and hopefully will encourage you to explore further the very rich literature that is emerging on mindfulness and mental health.

The following chapters will introduce you to the practice of mindfulness, so that you can experience first hand how it may strengthen you on your own particular recovery path. Mindfulness sounds like a pretty simple idea, but its power to change and transform your life is only revealed through practice.

The exercises you will be introduced to are the same methods that people all over the world are practising daily. I practise mindfulness myself, and find it to be immensely important and satisfying. Sometimes it's a sheer delight and other times, particularly when I am worried or upset about something, it is more challenging. But when I go back to the simple practices, which I will describe in the following chapters, I always find a way to be more comfortable with myself and to live each day more fully.

At the end of this book, I have included a list of books and resources that you may wish to explore, to learn more about mindfulness and to deepen your practice. I have also included websites of organisations and institutes that teach mindfulness courses and offer opportunities to practise with others and a CD of some of the exercises I have found to be most helpful in my personal life and in my teaching. You may want to listen to some of this CD while you read these chapters.

My hope is that, through mindfulness, you will learn to live more in the present and appreciate your life. When you encounter challenging situations in your life, as you inevitably will, my hope is that the practice of mindfulness will give you a safe way to relate to them rather than be discouraged by them. Above all, my hope is that you will discover through mindfulness that whatever pain and brokenness you experience in your life, they do not have the power to destroy you. You have a far greater power within you to heal and feel whole.

This quotation from a book of short stories by Barbara Kingsolver illustrates beautifully how she used mindfulness to climb out of a very dark place in her life:

Each one of us is called upon, probably many times, to start a new life. A frightening diagnosis, a marriage, a move, loss of a job or a limb or a loved one, a graduation, bringing a new baby home: it's impossible to think at first how this all will be possible. Eventually, what moves it all forward is the subterranean ebb and flow of being alive among the living.

In my own worst seasons I've come back from the colourless world of despair by forcing myself to look hard, for a long time, at a single glorious thing: a flame of red geranium outside my bedroom window. And then another: my daughter in a yellow dress. And another: the perfect outline of a full, dark sphere behind the crescent moon. Until I learned to be in love with my life again. Like a stroke victim retraining new parts of the brain to grasp lost skills, I have taught myself joy, over and over again.

Barbara Kingsolver, *High Tide in Tucson: Essays from Now or Never*

Summary

The real challenge facing someone who has recovered from an experience of depression is to learn to live with themselves in a way that reduces their likelihood of relapse. Mindfulness has a particular role in supporting our recovery and in helping us to weather the difficulties we encounter in our lives. It teaches us to steady ourselves in the present moment when we feel stressed. It grounds us and helps us to see more clearly what is happening, without being frightened or becoming overwhelmed. Research has shown again and again that mindfulness can protect many people from repeatedly relapsing into depression. Through mindfulness, we learn to appreciate positive experiences in our lives that can support our recovery, to heal places in our hearts where we may have been wounded, and to find the strength in ourselves to face situations where we feel threatened and vulnerable.

Message in a bottle

Mindfulness teaches you to relate
to your pain rather
than react to it.

CHAPTER 9

Learning to be mindful

A former student sent me a photograph that, for her, captured the experience of mindfulness. In the photograph, her child of 10 months, Michael, is sitting on a beach and experiencing for the first time the sensation of sand running through his fingers. His attention is completely in the present moment and his expression reveals how captivated he is by this sensation.

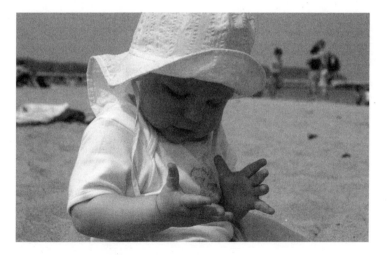

This photo expresses some key truths about mindfulness:
* We are mindful when we are present to what is happening in our lives.

- Mindfulness is a natural inborn skill in human beings. It is about returning to what is most natural for us.
- Because we live our lives with very little awareness of the richness and subtleties of the present moment, we need to practise this skill.
- To develop our capacity to be mindful, we need to bring this practice into our most basic everyday activities including resting, walking, breathing, sensing and listening.
- The goal of mindfulness is to live life more fully, to appreciate moments of our lives that all too easily pass us by.

You already have within yourself the capacity to be mindful. You can recover this capacity every time you choose to relate to this moment and whatever it holds for you, with kindness and with an open heart.

The exercises given over the next few chapters are simple 'practices' that can strengthen and deepen your capacity to be mindful. Try out these practices, one at a time. Give yourself as much time as you need to be comfortable with a particular practice before you proceed to the next. Don't try to take on too much, too fast. Stay within your limits, because if you honour your limits, they will naturally expand with your practice. Trust this process, don't push yourself. Don't be demoralised if your practice doesn't seem to 'work' for you. Accept what happens, whatever happens. Acceptance of your experience, as it is happening, is the very essence of mindfulness.

Being mindful of the present moment

The practice of resting, of stopping is crucial. If we cannot rest, it is because we have not stopped. We have continued to run. We began to run a long time ago. We even continue to run in our sleep.

Thich Nhat Hanh, *The Path of Emancipation*, p. 21

Rest is the basis of healing. When we allow our minds and bodies to settle, when we breathe in and out mindfully, we calm down and give ourselves a chance to heal. This is an act of kindness towards ourselves when we are feeling distressed or overwhelmed. It is also an expression of deep trust. When we are mindful, we create the conditions for our bodies and minds to heal and we trust that we have within us the capacity to heal.

Try stopping whatever you are doing and bring your attention to whatever is happening for you in this moment. Listen to the different sounds you can hear, coming at you from near and far. Notice how they weave in and out of each other, one sound standing out in the moment, another a moment later.

Notice the different colours and shapes around you, feel the air as it touches your skin and smell the different smells that you can pick up, both those that are subtle and those that are strong.

Notice the way your attention moves between the outer world and your inner world. Let your awareness flow between these worlds, without forcing anything.

Notice how easy it is to become caught up in some story in your mind that takes you away from the present moment and fills you with different feelings: 'This is boring', 'This is interesting, I remember reading something about this once'. See if you can gently notice your mind weaving some story or other, and then gently bring your attention back to a simple awareness of the sounds, colours and shapes around you.

To pay attention to whatever is unfolding in your life right now is more difficult than it sounds, partly because whenever we stop, we initially feel afraid. Our mind becomes crowded quickly, with thoughts that warn us that it's not safe to do this, that we should distract ourselves in some way by doing something that will take us away from this moment. To be present to what is happening, we have to learn to steady ourselves and be still. We use our breath to help us to calm down and rest in the present moment. Paying attention to the rhythm of our in-breath and our out-breath is the most basic and most important exercise in the practice of mindfulness.

Exercise one: Creating a safe place

Taking the time to stop, to rest and to be open to whatever is going on in your life can feel strange in the beginning. You may have been living your life in a different way for so long, running from one activity to the next, and trying so hard not to think about the things in your life that upset you, so it can feel a little unnerving to change. Mindfulness is not about gritting your teeth and making yourself change. It is a much more gentle activity than that. It also requires a great deal of patience, kindness and self-compassion.

What you are trying to do is create a safe place in yourself where you can settle down, and be grounded and open to your experience. As you learn to do this, you will be able to invite into that place whatever thoughts and feelings may be troubling you.

The practice of mindfulness always begins with making the place you are in a safe place, where you can become grounded. Wherever you are, at any given time, can be safe, when you bring your attention to that place and choose to be there. It is possible to practise mindfulness anywhere – for example, in a supermarket, in a police van, or in a boardroom – provided you become aware of where you are and you choose to be there.

To learn how to be mindful in this way, set aside a little time each day to practise. An athlete doesn't wait until the day of a competition to get fit; he or she will practise quietly in the gym or the local park, building their fitness without too much stress or pressure. Mindfulness is a capacity that you can also strengthen by practising alone or with others, so that when you really need it in the heat of a crisis, it is available to you.

Choose a place in your home, which you can make your 'safe' place. It could be a corner of your living room, a chair by the window in your bedroom, or any space in your home that is reasonably quiet, and where you are unlikely to be interrupted. Give yourself time to settle into this place until you are comfortable and alert. It may help to sit in an upright position, to open your chest, and to relax your arms and shoulders. Rest your hands on your lap and close your eyes if this feels natural for you. Alternatively you can focus your gaze on a spot on the floor a few feet in front of you.

Let your attention move through your body, from your head to your toes, and then allow it to settle on the rhythm of your breath. Find where it is easiest for you to follow your in-breath and your out-breath. It may be in the rise and fall of your belly or your chest; or it may be that you can follow it most easily by keeping your attention on the sensation of air moving in and out of your nostrils. Focus your attention wherever you find it easiest to stay with your breathing.

Follow your in-breath as it passes into your body and follow your out-breath as it passes out of your body. With each in-breath say to yourself, 'Breathing in, I know I am breathing in'; with each out-breath say, 'Breathing out, I know I am breathing out.' After a short while, you can shorten these phrases to 'in' with each in-breath and 'out' with each out-breath. This basic practice of mindfulness is called 'In–Out'.

Breathe naturally, don't worry about breathing deeply or breathing slowly. Whatever way you are breathing right now is just perfect. As you stay with each breath, you will notice that it naturally slows down and deepens. Your breath is the door through which you come home to yourself and rest in the present moment. By becoming aware of the rhythm of your in-breath and your out-breath, you bring your attention back to the present moment and connect with your body.

Become aware of the space around you. This is the place that your life has brought you to. It is your safe place. Imagine yourself as a mountain, strong and powerful, stable and still. And say to yourself: 'This is where I am now, this is where I am safe', 'This is where I stop running and come home to myself', 'This is where I choose to be'. Repeat any or all of these phrases to yourself and allow your body to settle into this place.

You may notice that, sooner or later, your attention drifts away from your breath, as your mind becomes distracted by some thought or feeling or sound. Don't be surprised by this. This is what your mind does, and it's been doing this for years.

When you notice your mind wandering, just smile. And then, as best you can, gently escort your attention back to your breath. If your attention wanders away from your breath a thousand times, gently escort your attention back to your breath a thousand times.

Enjoy your breathing. It is what keeps you alive. It works all by itself without you doing anything to make it work. If you have ever been unable to breathe for any reason, you will know what a wonderful gift it is just to be able to breathe in and breathe out naturally.

Your breath is a resting place that you can return to anytime, whatever is happening in you or around you. Becoming mindful of your breathing steadies your attention and anchors you in your body. Your worries and your fears will pull you constantly into the past or into the future. Your breath brings you back to your safe place in the present. When you are tired of being pulled here, there and everywhere by your mind, it's good to find a place where you can rest.

Reflecting on this experience

With practise, this exercise becomes easier and very enjoyable. But in the beginning it can be difficult. Mostly people find it hard because they try to 'make it work', they try to 'control' their breathing and 'stop' their mind wandering. They believe they have to do it in a certain way to 'get it right'. What they learn through practise is that they don't have to control anything; they simply have to enjoy breathing.

> As long as our breathing feels pleasant, we know that we are not working or manipulating it. Please pay attention to the effect of your in-breath and your out-breath on your body. If your breathing continues to give you pleasure, then you are doing it correctly.
>
> Thich Nhat Hanh, *The Path of Emancipation*, p. 150

When you breathe in a mindful way, you are not 'working on' your breath. You are actually trying to allow your breath to breathe. If your breath is short, you allow it to be short; if your breath is long, you allow it to be long.

As you bring awareness to your breathing, without trying to change it in any way, the rhythm of your breathing will naturally slow and deepen.

The instruction to smile whenever you notice your mind wandering may strike you as somewhat 'cheesy' but there is some wisdom behind it. Thich Nhat Hanh points out that there are about 300 muscles in the face. Every time we get angry, worried or afraid, these muscles tense up. If we allow ourselves to smile lightly as we breathe in and breathe out, we relax hundreds of muscles in our face. Smiling also saves us from taking ourselves too seriously.

Practising mindfulness at home

Take some time each day to practise this first exercise. In the beginning, you might decide to practise for three to five minutes. This is fine. As you grow stronger in the practice, you might want to increase the time you spend, particularly as you add in some of the practices described later (mindfulness of your body, feelings and thoughts). You may discover that practising for 10–20 minutes is what it takes to give you the time you need to really settle in to your safe place.

I find it helpful to have a clock within easy view when I practise. I decide on exactly how long I will practise before I start. I look at my clock and pick a 'finish time'. I settle into my safe place and stay there until I reach that time. I don't expect to feel any particular way or to achieve any particular kind of experience. I just do it and trust that by taking this time to practise, I will become more grounded in myself and live the day ahead of me with a little more awareness and appreciation.

When you approach your practice without any particular agenda or expectation, you may be surprised by what does happen. When you have been practising for a number of weeks, your practice can change the way you feel, give you greater clarity about what's important in your life, and enable creative solutions to emerge spontaneously to problems that you have been unable to resolve.

Sometimes when you practise, nothing much seems to happen. You will have days when it may be particularly hard to keep your attention on your breathing. In a practice session of 15 minutes, you may only manage to be present to yourself for one breath only. But that moment is worth a lot. And your efforts to be present to yourself, despite all the distractions, make it more likely that you will feel alive and alert in the day ahead.

Practising mindfulness 'on the go'

There are many ways that you can drop in on your breath throughout the day as you move around from one activity to another. The practice of 'dropping in' on your breath will help you to be more present to what you are doing and calms your mind.

- **Breathing as you wash your hands**: As you wash your hands bring your attention to your in-breath and to your out-breath. As you breathe, feel the sensation of the water pouring over your hands and allow your attention to stay with this pleasurable sensation until you have completed washing.
- **Breathing as you listen to music:** Follow your breath as you listen to a piece of music, keeping some part of your awareness on the music and some part of your awareness on your breath. Enjoy the music, feel its passion and really listen to the different elements of sound that work together to create its impact.
- **Breathing while carrying on a conversation:** It is so easy to become distracted when listening to a friend, even when what they are sharing is important to you. Drop in on your breath and use your breath to bring you back to the present moment so that you can really hear what they are saying.

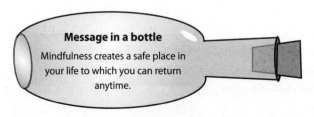

Message in a bottle
Mindfulness creates a safe place in your life to which you can return anytime.

CHAPTER 10

Relating mindfully to your body

S ometimes your body can feel like a stranger to you. You may not like it and wish it was a different shape or size. You may even wish at times that you didn't have to deal with it at all. When you feel this way about your body, it's easy to distance yourself from all the sensations and feelings it holds. Breathing mindfully can bring you back to your body, so that you can listen to what it needs, and to what it may be trying to communicate to you.

> The value of cultivating mindfulness is not just a matter of getting more out of sunsets. When unawareness dominates the mind, all our decisions and actions are affected by it. Unawareness can keep us from being in touch with our body, its signals and messages.
>
> Jon Kabat-Zinn, *Full Catastrophe Living*

Learning to connect with and listen to your body is the second exercise in the practice of mindfulness. Mindfulness of the body invites you to consider a different way of relating to whatever sensations, tensions and feelings may be there. When you become aware of these sensations, you may want to push them away or to 'think' them away. Mindfulness, in contrast, invites you to notice where you may be holding tension in your body, and to gently soften in those places. Notice what you may be trying to block out or push away and invite these sensations into your safe place. Connect with your body so that you can listen to it and be guided by its signals.

Exercise two: Relating kindly to your body

This exercise builds on Exercise One, which you have been practising. When you have found your safe place and settled into an easy rhythm of following your in-breath and your out-breath, you may notice that you naturally become aware of your body. As you do, try saying the following:

> Breathing in, I am aware of my body
> Breathing out, I calm my body
> Aware of my body …
> Calm my body …

This exercise enables you to come back to your body and to attend to it with kindness and gentleness. When you experience your body, you may become aware of where you are holding tension; a tightness in your shoulders, a heaviness in your chest or your stooped posture, may each signal different ways that you are tensing and contracting your body.

> Breathing in, I am aware of my body
> Breathing out, I calm my body
> Aware …
> Calm …

Don't expect your body to change quickly just because you are finally paying attention to it. You may have rejected it many times in the past and it's hard for your body to trust that you won't abandon it again. You may need to spend time holding it in awareness before it can feel safe enough to let go of any tension and relax.

Extend your safe place exercise to incorporate the lines above and let it be part of whatever practice routine you are developing for yourself.

Exercise three: Scanning your entire body

Bring your awareness to every part of your body, starting with your feet and working your way gradually up through your whole body.

This method is called the body scan because you focus the full energy of your attention on each part of your body, much like an X-ray machine might scan each part of the body. It generally takes 15–20 minutes to complete this body scan exercise slowly and it can be done most easily if you are lying down. If you do lie down, cover yourself with a rug to keep warm. I have included a guided body scan exercise on the CD that comes with this book.

Reflections on these exercises

When we stop and reconnect with our bodies, we often become aware of pain and tension that we have been avoiding. This can frighten us, because we fear that connecting with whatever sensations may be there will make us feel worse than we already do. So, once again, the way we relate to whatever we discover in our bodies is critically important. Thich Nhat Hanh describes mindfulness as a way of 'holding' our bodies in our awareness as a mother might hold a child:

You breathe in and embrace each part of your body with mindfulness, like a mother holding her baby in her tender arms. And smile to it. This is very healing, very important.

Thich Nhat Hanh, *The Path of Emancipation*, p. 37

Mindfulness brings our attention to where there is tension and pain in our bodies and enables us to stay with our bodily experience and release that tension. Sometimes we need the help of a therapist or mindfulness teacher to make it safe for us to connect with our bodies and let go the tension we find there.

Homework: Tuning into how your body feels

In the week ahead, find a quiet place and take time to create your safe space as we did in Chapter 9. Extend the 'breathing' exercise very slightly by including in it an awareness of your body.

Breathing in, I know that I am breathing in
Breathing out, I know that I am breathing out
In …
Out …
Breathing in, I am aware of my body
Breathing out, I calm my body
Aware …
Calm …

In addition, set aside some additional time to try out the body scan exercise. This is very much a key exercise in building up your capacity to be mindful. You will find that if you practise this exercise, it will be much easier to stay in touch with the 'signals and messages' your body is sending you.

There are also simple ways that you can come back to your body as you go through the day. Below are a few you might want to try in the coming week.

Being aware of the position your body is in

Whether you are standing, sitting, stretching or lying down, bring your attention back to your body and notice how it feels. For example, be aware of your body as you bend over to pick up something. Notice the different muscles that are involved in helping to accomplish this task.

If you practise yoga, or any kind of stretching exercises, pay close attention to the sensations you feel in your body as you move and stretch. Notice the difference in your body, before and after a stretch; if you experience some pain towards the end of a stretch, bring your full awareness to that pain and see if you can relate to it with kindness before you release your body from that position.

When you lie down at night, check in with your body before you fall asleep; move your awareness from your toes to your head and back again, being thankful for all the ways your body has supported you in living through the day.

Being aware of restlessness in your body

Notice those times when your body feels agitated and restless. This energy may feel hard to contain. You want to move around to dissipate this energy. It's hard to relax, to feel at peace. Acknowledge the energy of restlessness and accept it: 'Breathing in, I know I am restless; breathing out, I accept my restlessness.' This may be all you can do right now. Accept it and be gentle with it. Walk around if you need to. Notice how walking slowly can help to release the energy of restlessness or make it easier to bear.

Calming your body

To give any activity your full attention, it helps to calm your body. However, before you can calm your body, you first have to stop and remember it is there. Try to stop whatever you are doing at different points in the day and say to yourself: 'Breathing in, I am aware of my body, breathing out I smile at my body.'

It helps to identify routine events in your everyday life that can serve as reminders to stop and calm your body. A red traffic light can be an annoyance, but it can also be a reminder to stop, breathe and calm your body. When a phone rings, it can be a reminder to take one breath and calm yourself before answering. In the short gap between one meeting ending and another beginning, allow yourself to come back to your body, to breathe and to ground yourself.

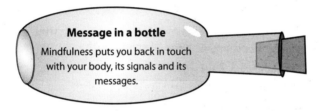

Message in a bottle

Mindfulness puts you back in touch with your body, its signals and its messages.

CHAPTER 11

Relating mindfully to your emotions

If you embrace a minor pain with mindfulness, it will be transformed in a few minutes. Just breathe in and out, and smile at it. But when you have a block of pain that is stronger, more time is needed. Practice sitting and walking meditation while you embrace your pain in mindfulness, and sooner or later, it will be transformed. If you have increased the quality of your mindfulness through the practice, the transformation will be quicker. When mindfulness embraces pain it begins to penetrate and transform it, like sunshine penetrating a flower bud and helping it blossom. When mindfulness touches something beautiful it reveals its beauty. When it touches something painful it transforms and heals it.

Thich Nhat Hahn, *Touching Peace*

I n Part Two of this book, we looked at some of the ways we can recover from depression through reaching out to others for support, structuring our day, becoming aware of self-defeating thoughts and beliefs that are associated with depression, and not buying into their negative thought patterns. But even when our mood lifts, our bodies continue to carry the memory of the hurts, losses and disappointments that we have experienced in our lives. And our mind still carries a tendency to react to new and remembered sorrows where we turn against ourselves and believe we are to blame for the way we feel.

Recovery implies that we gradually become open to our sorrows, and recognise that they are part of who we are. In this way, we allow disowned parts of ourselves room to breathe and to heal. We become less divided in ourselves, we feel stronger, and we gradually recover a sense of ourselves as people who are capable of growing and changing in positive ways.

Mary was a woman who had many severe episodes of depression. Her psychiatrist had recommended mindfulness to her but she knew nothing about it. I started to explain it to her and she became noticeably tense and uneasy. She was full of fear that if she were to acknowledge painful feelings inside her, she would relapse into depression.

I asked her if she had an image of where her life was at that precise moment. She had recently recovered from a severe bout of depression. She described her recovery as having walked through a door to a much calmer and gentler place in her life. 'But', she said, 'the door is still open.' She feared she could be sucked back into the darkness of depression at any time.

I noticed that as she described this image she became calmer. She agreed with my observation and I asked her why she thought her mood had shifted so significantly. 'Because I know where I am,' she replied. Her words were an elegant explanation of mindfulness; in acknowledging to herself where she was and in allowing herself to be there, she experienced a moment of mindfulness.

Knowing where you are at any moment in time is the most important step you will take in learning to take care of yourself. If you are angry and you can see that you are angry, that is a start. At least then you are much less likely to act on this anger in ways that may surprise and startle you. Mindfulness is about taking time to know where you are, even though this may be painful. It may not be easy to stand in the place you are in right now, to feel the feelings that are there, but it is the only real place you can stand.

If you can look at your distress directly, you can find a way out of it. If you run away from your feelings and refuse to accept that they are there, you will never have a chance to move beyond them. By changing the way you relate to your inner experience, you open up possibilities to change your experience.

One of the ways that the experience of depression offers us a chance to grow is by bringing us closer to feelings and emotions from which we have spent our whole lives running. Through our struggle with depression, we become alert to ways in which our mind and our heart have become disconnected. Before depression, we may have relied heavily on our mind to keep certain feelings and memories at a safe distance. We lived in our heads and became strangers to our hearts. When we became depressed, it was harder to keep our feelings hidden. Our hearts may have opened and brought into our awareness feelings of pain and grief that we had suppressed for a long time.

The practice of mindfulness gives us a way to befriend our emotions and not to be afraid of them. Without a living relationship with our emotions, we never know where we are and we experience our lives as empty. When we learn to live mindfully with our emotions, we stay in touch with who we are, and we give our wounds a chance to heal.

Exercise four: Creating a safe space and making friends with your emotions

Sit quietly and comfortably. Bring your awareness back to your breath and to your body. Feel yourself settle into your safe space. Take as much time as you need to slow down, and feel grounded and strong. Repeat as often as you wish any or all of the following phrases: 'This is my safe place', ' This is where I sit', 'This is where I am safe'.

Notice whatever sensations may be present in your body and

bring your attention to them. Are there particular feelings that accompany these sensations? Do not push away these feelings. Meet them with warmth and compassion as you would a lost child. Assure these feelings that you want to get to know them. Tell them that you regret the years you have spent trying to run from them and deny they were there. Now you are going to listen to them, to allow them room to breathe and to connect with them.

Allow your heart to open and give it whatever time it needs to realise that you are not going to attack it for feeling whatever it feels. Feel your heart's energies as they move through your body. Notice where in your body you can detect emotion. Become aware of the way you may contract your muscles in those parts of your body, as though you were trying to protect yourself and keep certain feelings at bay. See if you can relax your body in those places where you are holding tension and give your emotions room to breathe. Let go of the urge to change how you feel. Your task is not to change your feelings, but to open to them.

Allow your feelings to come and go as they please. Notice how they ebb and flow when you don't try to block them. Notice subtle ways their intensity changes and how one feeling is replaced by another.

Relate to each feeling that arises with respect and kindness. Hold it in your awareness as a mother might hold a troubled child in her arms. Your soothing presence is all it needs. If you find yourself losing touch with your safe place and becoming carried away by these feelings, go back to your breath and take whatever time you need to recover your peace and steady yourself.

When you are ready, thank your feelings for revealing themselves to you. Finish this exercise and stand up.

Reflection on this exercise

A common reaction to noticing the presence of some unpleasant feeling is to become caught up in some story or other about why you feel this way, how unfair it is that you feel upset, or how 'weak' you are for feeling so vulnerable. Whatever you are feeling, there is a very good reason for it. But, for now, try to let go of the story you tell yourself about these feelings and see if you can sense where they are and how exactly they are making their presence known in your body.

Being mindful enables you to be aware of thoughts and behaviours that can be triggered by unpleasant feelings: 'I can't stand this', 'I must stop this feeling', etc. Mindful awareness makes it possible to let go of these thoughts gradually, or at least turn down the volume on whatever storyline is emerging, and be present to the way you experience these feelings in your body.

Your feelings are expressions of the energy within you. It is only when you react against these energies with stories and fantasies, that their presence feels thick and heavy. Holding them in your awareness with kindness and compassion enables these feelings to unfold in a different way and to resolve in their own time.

See if you can let go of the stories for now, turn down the volume on your thinking mind and stay with what you are feeling with an attitude of openness and acceptance. Feel what you are feeling and let it be, without judging it as either good or bad.

Our first encounter with our emotions, when we begin to be mindful of them, can be humbling and frightening. The energies of our buried emotions may be very strong. When we accept them and allow them room to breathe, we may feel like we're 'falling apart'. But what may actually be happening is that we are finally 'coming together'. When we anchor ourselves in our safe place, we allow ourselves to feel the rawness of our fear, the grief we experienced when we lost someone we loved, the anger we felt at being abandoned or abused. For the first time, we are in a position to acknowledge these emotions and to honour them. They show us that whatever happened to cause us to feel this way was something that really mattered to us. And because we have never appreciated this, we have spent our whole life feeling that there must be something wrong with us.

Pain can be hard to bear, but it can clarify so much. We can feel like we are dying, but the part of us that is dying is often the scared defensive part of us that has served its time and now needs to be released. Something deeper in us is trying to come alive: a more connected grounded person who feels compassion for themself and for others, someone who may want to cry, and someone who may want to laugh. After years of feeling that there was something 'wrong' and hiding from others, we can finally feel free. We see now that we don't have to 'be reasonable', 'be good' and 'keep a lid on our feelings' all of the time.

If you love someone, there is no greater gift you can give them than that of being present to them. Your presence and your acceptance of who they are and whatever they are feeling in that particular moment can soothe them and strengthen them. You don't even have to say anything; your silent presence can be immensely healing for them. Relating mindfully to your feelings works in the same way. It is the practice of being present to whatever you are feeling, right here and right now. Breathing in and breathing out, you commit to being there for yourself and accepting whatever you are experiencing in this moment.

Equipped with mindfulness, we can go home safely and not be overwhelmed by our pain, sorrow, and depression. Going home mindfully, we can talk to our wounded child within using the following mantra: 'Darling, I have come home to you. I am here for you. I embrace you in my arms. I am sorry I have left you alone for a long time.'

Thich Nhat Hanh, *The Path of Emancipation*, p. 92

Being aware of whatever you are feeling and naming it tends to shift your feelings into a different space. When you move towards fear instead of running away from it, your feeling of dread may open into a feeling of sadness. You may feel suddenly alone, even though you are surrounded by others; you may see clearly as if for the very first time, that you have been running from fear all your life and you may finally realise how exhausting this has been. The key is to accept and allow yourself to feel whatever is there.

Taking time to notice the different feelings you have each day

If you are like most people who have experienced depression, you may be overly sensitive to 'bad' feelings and miss out on noticing moments where you actually feel good. Like the man who had a toothache and couldn't think of anything else when it was there. But when it was all over, he never noticed or appreciated how good it was to wake up every day without that ache.

Being mindful of your feelings and emotions does not mean that we should only focus on those that are painful or distressing. To build a stronger relationship with our emotions, it helps to take some time at the end of each day and reflect on the wide range of emotions you experienced that day, including those that were pleasant.

Savour those moments and be thankful for them. Think about moments when you felt compassion for others; think of the ways you were generous and giving to others; think of moments when you felt appreciation for something very simple in life; and when you responded with love in a natural spontaneous way.

Summary

These simple exercises have been shown to have a very positive effect on our immune system. We become more aware that we have a wide range of feelings, which come and go and change all the time. And we become more aware of the way our emotions can connect us with others, and enable us to share our lives with them.

Before we invite our painful feelings into our 'safe place', it helps to acknowledge the good feelings we have also experienced in the course of the day, even if they were brief and even if they weren't very strong in us. It is all too easy to become preoccupied with what is not working in our lives, to fixate on where we are in conflict within ourselves, and to lose sight of the bigger picture. Acknowledging positive experiences and pleasant feelings, opens out our awareness. Our awareness becomes more spacious and we can acknowledge our pain without feeling that life has completely forgotten us.

> Whatever problem, question, or confusion we have, whatever seems impossible in our lives, if we go towards it, see it, feel it and make a relationship with it, it can become our path to waking up and becoming whole.
>
> John Welwood, *Toward a Psychology of Awakening*

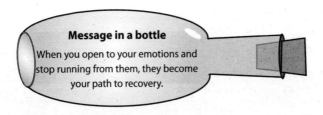

Message in a bottle

When you open to your emotions and stop running from them, they become your path to recovery.

CHAPTER 12

Relating mindfully to your thoughts

Sometimes it is pleasant to allow your mind to float to wherever it wants go, buffeted around by the breezes of memory and anticipation. This is certainly true when our thoughts and feelings are pleasant and when our future looks promising and full of possibilities. But what happens when our thoughts are not pleasant, when our mind becomes carried away on some thought safari that ends up in some familiar dark hole?

> I find it so hard to be with my thoughts, to be in my head that I haven't even been able to take a bath in years – I just can't be alone with my thoughts, I live in yesterdays and tomorrows. I hate meditation, but I need to slow my head down … to get myself into today.
>
> John, aged 33, participant on mindfulness-training course

It can be very hard to relax into your own company, because of the thoughts that arise in your mind. For people who have been depressed, these difficult thoughts often remind them of times in their lives when they were overcome by despair. These thoughts can also remind them of experiences in their lives that they would rather forget. How are we to find peace in ourselves to deal with these thoughts without being overwhelmed by them?

The gift of cognitive therapy is to show how powerfully our

thinking affects our mood. Whatever difficulties we encounter in our lives, it is the way in which we think about these events that influences how confident we feel to respond to them.

The thoughts we find more difficult are usually those where we make harsh self-judgments; thoughts that remind us of all the ways that we believe ourselves to be weak, shameful and unworthy. In Chapter 5, we explored some of the childhood roots of these thoughts and beliefs, and how they can be triggered by particular events in our lives. They never completely go away, but we can learn to stand back from them and see them for what they are.

Why do we entertain these self-attacking thoughts that seriously undermine our self-confidence? Sometimes it is because we feel that this will help us to 'get a grip' or to 'grow up' and to 'stop being such a baby'. Sometimes we resort to thinking this way because we believe it is the only way we can 'keep it together' in moments when we feel we are losing control over our lives.

The fact is, however, that these harsh thoughts deepen our distress rather than help us to deal with it. When we react to our pain with a barrage of self-criticism, we dig ourselves more deeply into the very hole from which we are trying to escape.

Cognitive therapy shows us a variety of ways to become aware of these thoughts, and to deal with them by writing them down and challenging them. Mindfulness goes one step further. It shows us how we can become aware of them, and allow them be present in our minds, without getting carried away by them. Relating mindfully to our thoughts means acknowledging them while staying rooted in our safe place. Mindfulness also shows us how to view these thoughts through the lens of self-compassion.

Let me give you a concrete example of how this worked for a group of people who had experienced many episodes of depression in their lives. Each person on our mindfulness training courses in St James's Hospital in Dublin was all too familiar with negative thoughts. In one of the classes, we invited them to reflect on an upsetting event they had experienced during the previous week and to write down whatever had passed through their minds at the time. Each of them wrote down a stream of negative thoughts at the beginning of the session and rated these on a 0–100 per cent scale to indicate how much they believed each thought.

We didn't talk about what they had written at that time. They set their thought records to one side and we continued the group with a series of mindful stretching and breathing exercises. After about 45 minutes, we invited the class to review what they had written and to re-rate how strongly they believed each of the negative thoughts they had written down.

There was a remarkable shift in their belief in these negative thoughts when they were re-rated. When we explored what had happened to bring about this change, the group described how following the mindfulness exercises meant they looked at their thoughts in a whole new way. They saw how hurtful these thoughts were, and remembered many times when these same thoughts had caused them to feel depressed in the past. But following their practise of mindfulness they saw these thoughts for what they were and these thoughts no longer had the same power over them. They also felt a compassion for themselves that they hadn't experienced before, because they appreciated that their pushing, fearful thoughts were coming from a place of hurt in themselves.

This experience reveals one of the ways that relating mindfully to our thoughts can make us less vulnerable to becoming depressed. Normally, when we experience our thoughts and emotions drawing us into a cycle that can lead to depression, we begin to struggle against them. While this is a natural reaction, it rarely works. What pulls us out of such a downturn in our mood is something much more subtle.

The practice of mindfulness shifts our consciousness to a deeper level and steadies us in that place. We see our life from a new perspective. Mindfulness doesn't make our negative thoughts go away; it creates a much larger frame of reference where we see our thoughts as a part of the story of our lives, but by no means the whole story. Mindfulness connects us with the much larger story of our lives where we feel connected to the world around us and to other people who also wrestle with similar pain and distress. It also encourages an attitude of compassion towards ourselves for all the ways we struggle, as best we can, to cope with the hurt and the pain we have known. It liberates us from the narrow identification of our lives with these destructive thoughts and opens our awareness to a much larger appreciation of how precious it is to be alive.

Exercise five: Relating mindfully to your negative thoughts

By now, the same message has been repeated over and over, that whenever you try to be mindful, you can expect that your mind will wander. You are all too aware of how painful some of your thoughts can be, and how easy it is to become carried away by them. In this exercise, you will be invited to look more closely at your thoughts and to see them for what they are: opinions, particular points of view and ideas that pass through your mind. They are thoughts rather than truths, and it is only when we buy into them that they can cause distress.

Returning to your 'safe place', settle yourself into a comfortable upright posture and take a few minutes to breathe mindfully and to bring your attention back to the present moment.

> Breathing in, I know I am breathing in
> Breathing out, I know I am breathing out
> In …
> Out …

Notice how your mind wanders and enables you to look at the particular thoughts that take your attention away from your breath. Some people find it helpful to imagine themselves sitting in a cinema, looking up at a giant blank screen. When a thought enters your mind, imagine it passing across the screen, as you sit there and watch.

Notice the different thoughts that arise in your mind. Are they encouraging or discouraging? Are they critical or shaming? Are they new or familiar thoughts? Notice the effect these thoughts have on your body and on your general mood. Notice how some of these thoughts are hurtful. Acknowledge whatever thoughts are there, and then gently bring your attention back to your breath. See your thoughts for what they are, but don't cling to them or try to do battle with them. Acknowledge them, and then let them go.

> Breathing in, I see how thinking distracts my mind
> Breathing out, I let go of my thoughts
> See my thoughts …
> Let go my thoughts …

Whenever your thoughts seem to be stealing you away, notice this happening, name what is happening by simply saying 'thinking' to yourself and bring your attention back to your breath. Take whatever time you need to settle back into your body, to feel grounded and steady.

Sometimes your thoughts have been triggered by some

problem that remains unresolved. If there is a specific problem that continues to distract you, acknowledge to yourself that this is a problem in your life that may require some attention. Agree to take some steps to address this problem later, but, for now, allow yourself to let it be and come back to your breath.

Naming themes and patterns

When it comes to negative thought patterns, spotting those that are most familiar to you and giving them a name can reduce the grip that they have over you. When you are breathing mindfully, and familiar thoughts distract you, see if you can find a word that captures the essence of what they are about. If you notice your thoughts have a critical theme to them, you might label this as 'my punishing mind' and let it go; similarly, you might label familiar thoughts as 'my fearful mind' or 'my bossy mind', 'my I'm-no-good mind', 'my I-can't-do-anything-right mind', 'my this-is-all-my fault-mind' and so on.

Notice how the thoughts and storylines that arise are the very ones that keep you stuck in your life and alienated from your true self. They tend to become activated by things that go wrong in your life, or by some perception you may have that wherever you are in your life, you should be somewhere else. Recognise that, in some ways, they are a habit you have developed through your life to cope with fear and disappointment. See them for what they are but do not imagine that what they are saying to you is true. You are doing the best you can in your life right now. You need encouragement and patience; you do not need the pain that these thoughts provoke in you – you have depths of strength and creativity that these particular thoughts know nothing about. As you practise this exercise, you will discover new depths in yourself. When your mind is settled, creative solutions to the problems you face can and will emerge.

Summary

When you overcome an episode of depression, another journey begins. This journey involves learning to deepen your awareness of your life as it unfolds, moment by moment, day by day. This awareness will help you to know where you are at any given time and to look after yourself. Deepening your awareness of what is happening in your life will also help you to live it more fully.

Recovery means finding a new way to relate to our thoughts and emotions. It invites us to make friends with our feelings gradually, to become open to our sorrows and to recognise that they are part of who we are. Recovery also requires that we become familiar with thought patterns that blame us for the way we feel. Our negative thoughts, and the destructive stories that we weave from them, are just one more example of how we struggle to make sense of our pain. Mindfulness gives us a way of holding our pain with compassion and enabling it to unfold in a different way.

Mindfulness is a skill that enables you to be aware without becoming overwhelmed. It teaches you a new way to relate to experiences in your life where you feel threatened and vulnerable. It also teaches you greater appreciation of those elements in your life that support you and bring you happiness.

This change of attitude towards difficult emotions and thoughts is fundamental to the practice of mindfulness. It is a way of living with ourselves that is captured in a poem by the 13th-century mystic, Rumi. Entitled 'Guest House', this poem captures the essence of how to relate mindfully to your thoughts and emotions.

> This being human is a Guest house
> Every morning a new arrival.

A joy, a depression, a meanness
Some momentary awareness comes
As an unexpected visitor.
Welcome and entertain them all!
Even if they are a crowd of sorrows,
Who violently sweep your house
empty of its furniture,

Still, treat each guest honourably.
He may be clearing you out
for some new delight.

The dark thought, the shame, the malice.
Meet them at the door laughing
And invite them in.

Be grateful for whoever comes
Because each has been sent
as a guide from beyond.

Message in a bottle

Mindfulness shows you how to accept
your thoughts without becoming
lost in them.

CHAPTER 13

Living mindfully

Let's lie down
Close our eyes
And listen to the music of the sun
To the grass singing
Let words have a rest
And speech a little siesta

Nazand Begikhani

When we are mindful, we connect deeply with the present moment. We see what is around us, we are in touch with our bodies and we are present to whatever is happening. We disengage from thinking about life and we live it.

When we drink a cup of coffee, we feel the shape of the cup we are holding in our hands, we smell the aroma of the coffee, we sip and taste its unique flavour. When we catch our mind drifting away into regrets about the past or worries about the future, we simply bring our awareness back to what is happening right here, right now. We are present; we feel alive.

When we bring an attitude of curiosity and kindness to whatever is happening, we notice that our awareness deepens in a very short time; we feel connected to what is happening in us and around us. We come home to ourselves and touch what is most real in our lives.

As I sat here earlier this morning, I looked across the river below me and watched a heron standing on the far bank. It was very still; and as I watched it with curiosity, I became quieter within myself.

Behind the heron was a high stone wall. And behind the wall, there was an apartment block, with a large steel gate protecting its entrance.

My attention was drawn to this gate as an ambulance, its lights flashing, quietly pulled up outside it. A person appeared and let the ambulance inside. Two men climbed up some steps into the apartment block and reappeared minutes later carrying someone on a stretcher. The heron turned its head at the sound they made; it looked up in their direction, and kept on looking until the ambulance drove away.

I felt very connected to the heron and to the little drama that was unfolding before my eyes. Somehow it made me aware of how fragile our lives are. At some point in all our lives, something happens that takes us by surprise and reminds us of our fragility. The heron and I were both witnesses to a moment of fragility in someone's life. His or her pain did not go unnoticed. In some way, the three of us were connected in that moment, and, then, it passed.

We paint the story of our lives on a very large canvas, but we can only live our lives one moment at a time. Mindfulness is the energy of attention that we bring to each moment. When we are mindful, we are present and attentive to what we are doing, the person we are with, the setting we are in. When we are mindful, we invest ourselves in what we are doing; however simple it is, however complex it may be. We can be mindful of chopping an onion, closing a door. We can be mindfully present to someone when we listen to them as they share with us some experience in their lives.

The opposite of living mindfully is rushing from one activity to the next, performing each one on automatic pilot, our minds always somewhere else. We skim over the surface of experience, rarely getting to savour it. We speed-date reality and hurry through each day, barely noticing what we are doing and always asking, 'What's next?'

Living constantly on automatic pilot can leave us feeling empty and driven. When we stop, we can feel uneasy in our own company. We look to the future, our next project or some new distraction, to save us from ourselves. Time becomes our enemy. We complain that we never have enough time but, when we do, we try to 'kill time' by watching TV, picking up the phone or rushing around. Our life can become a series of attempts to escape our own company. We pay little attention to our bodies, our feelings and our deeper concerns. Until it is too late, when something goes wrong and we wonder why we didn't see it coming.

If we choose to live mindfully, we do so because we want to be freer in our lives. We are tired of being driven by our fears and misperceptions; we want to connect with the person we really are and to live more authentically in the world. We want to make choices that lead somewhere new, rather than be driven by habit and compulsions that take us back into territory that is familiar and safe; we want to know more clearly what is true for us, so that we can speak to others in our own voice and we want to be genuinely present to others and listen to what they are trying to say to us with their voice.

We want to wake up from the dreamlike trance we have mistaken for reality, to realise that things don't always have to be the way they have been: that we don't have to keep looking into other people's eyes for stop and go signals; that we don't always have to run and hide every time we feel hurt and afraid; that we have options about how we choose to live. The only thing we owe to ourselves and the world is that we exercise our options, as mindfully as we can, to the best of our ability.

The benefits of practice

Mindfulness has a role in recovery because it teaches you how to live with yourself; it shows you a way to listen to and take care of yourself. As you learn to stop and take time to be mindful, this practice gradually changes how you experience your life. You may find that you are much more open and aware of very simple things in your life that make up your day and help to give it meaning.

Mindfulness helps you to be at ease with yourself. You learn to be at home with your own thoughts and feelings. Your mind settles and you become less dependent on things outside yourself to find peace. Mindfulness enables you to appreciate and enjoy the creativity of your own mind. You learn to think your own thoughts, to reach certain conclusions that are in line with your own deeper intelligence, and to live your life in a way that is right for you. You gradually discover a new freedom in yourself to be who you are, and to speak with your own unique voice. You find an inner strength not from what you can get out of things and people, but from knowing what it is that you want to give to life and to others.

Depression stems from all the hidden sadness, hurt and guilt that we have shut off within ourselves. Healing is about choosing to listen to these feelings and finding ways to accept and take care of the hurts we've experienced. Sitting with calm awareness, we can create space for these disowned parts of ourselves; we can finally give them room to breathe. At some point, we come to a realisation that we want to stop running, that we want to learn to be with ourselves and make room for the different parts of ourselves that are real, so that we can be who we are and enjoy this precious life that is ours.

I learned most about the value of mindfulness from people who have participated in the courses I have run at an inner-city psychiatric hospital in Dublin. These people came to mindfulness training with histories of severe and enduring mental health difficulties. For them, mindfulness was not simply some kind of an add-on to their lives, like a second TV or an iPod, they participated because they wanted to find a way of living with difficulties that no treatment had resolved. They took to learning mindfulness as though their lives depended on it, and in many cases it did.

One of these people was a man named Frank. Aged 37, he had already been admitted to a psychiatric hospital on 20 different occasions. He had been given every kind of diagnosis in his time, but depression and psychosis were at the heart of most of them. He asked to join the group but I wasn't at all sure at first if it would be of any benefit to him. Whilst there was a growing literature at the time that clearly showed that mindfulness-based cognitive therapy was effective in preventing relapse into depression, there was, as yet, no evidence showing that it could help people with psychosis. But Frank was insistent and I agreed we would give it a try.

Being a devout Catholic, Frank would pray daily for 20 minutes and then do a further 20 minutes' practice of mindfulness meditation at a later point in the day. He believed in the practice, but he was never sure that mindfulness would be as acceptable to God as conventional prayer.

One day, half-jokingly over the tea break, I asked him if he was getting anything at all out of the practice. He seemed surprised by my question and wondered why I would even ask it of him. He told me that since beginning the practice of mindfulness, his medication had been reduced to half the dose it had been, he had moved out of the hospital into independent accommodation, he was volunteering two days a week at a centre for people with mental health problems and he had taken up an Open University course.

One experience he described convinced me more than any other that this practice of mindfulness was working for him. I am relaying this story to answer the question that is most commonly asked of me, by people who feel that I may be asking too much of them to believe that this practice of mindfulness could help them with severe emotional upset: 'What good can it do to try to be aware of my feelings, in the here and now, when all I am feeling is distress?'

The previous week, Frank had been travelling alone on a commuter train, sitting quietly lost in thought. Something distracted him and he looked across the carriage at his fellow passengers. He saw blue rays of light coming from the eyes of two of his fellow passengers and he became highly alarmed. At that precise point, he recognised he was in the grip of a panic attack and started to focus on his breathing.

> I closed my eyes and went back to my breath. And when I did I became aware of how totally stressed I was everywhere in my body. I realised that I had been trying to do too much. I had got so worked up about my work and my course that I was over-stressed. I realised that what I thought I had seen was simply a hallucination. After a few minutes of breathing, I opened my eyes and the blue lights were gone from the people sitting opposite me.

Many times in the past Frank had had similar experiences. He explained that, without the practice, he would have run to another carriage where he would have most likely seen many more people with blue lights streaming from their eyes. And at that point, he would have left the train and probably kept running until he got home. There, he would have tried to hide from the dangers he perceived to be lurking around every corner, until eventually he would have been admitted to hospital.

Frank's story of recovery from a brief psychotic episode illustrates the power of mindfulness to save him from spiralling into a complete breakdown. His awareness of being upset, his choice to return to a safe place in himself and take time to breathe and ground himself had enabled him to steer himself gently out of difficulty. Mindfulness served as a protective factor in that moment and it continued to serve him until his death a year later from pancreatic cancer. Before his death, he co-led a mindfulness training group with me for people who were attempting to recover from severe multiple addictions. That group was the first systematic study of mindfulness with addiction in Ireland. Although it was just one group, the results were very positive and it has inspired several applications of mindfulness training in the field of addiction. The study – the DEORA Mindfulness Programme (Bates & Scanlan, 2008) – is dedicated to Frank's memory.

Building the practice of mindfulness into your daily routine

Many of the practices described in these chapters can be fitted into your normal day, whenever you catch yourself being carried away by thoughts and worries, and when you want to come back to the present moment and steady yourself. The Safe Place exercise is generally one that people prefer to practise in the morning, usually after a number of stretching exercises (mindful stretches, yoga) to 'wake up' the body and give you more energy, although it can of course be practised at any time of day that suits you.

Take some time every day to learn to go back to your safe place and attend to your breathing mindfully, and connect with your deep inner strength. There will always be thoughts and bodily sensations that emerge and cause you stress, but as you practise mindfulness, what begins to happen is that your capacity to note these and to attend to them, with kindness and appreciation, becomes steadier. And with that steadiness comes a deeper understanding and insight into those elements and experiences in your life that keep repeating over and over. Understanding, along with insight, frees you from automatic patterns of reacting to your inner world by trying to avoid it, or by becoming caught up in self-defeating behaviours. Being able to catch yourself slipping into the behaviours enables you to ground yourself in the present and make some new choices about how you might wish to live your life.

Summary

Mindfulness is one element, or one expression, of a general philosophy of what it takes to become human. Mindfulness comes from spiritual traditions in the East and West that articulated a number of elements required for people to discover their true selves and find their place in the world. All of these philosophies recognise that it is easy for humans to get it wrong, to lose their way and become alienated from others.

The practice of mindfulness has come to us through these different spiritual traditions, but this does not mean that you are expected or required to sign up to some particular religion or school of thought. Mindfulness works best, however, when it's undertaken as part of a commitment to take more care of yourself and to grow in your appreciation and respect for all living things.

Daily practice of mindfulness can be important to support and strengthen your recovery. If you are someone who is vulnerable to feeling depressed, the exercises described in these chapters can help you to catch the early warning signs of a change in your mood. These practices embody a philosophy of compassion and kindness. They have emerged from ancient traditions that valued life and appreciated that both people and the natural world are dependent on one another to survive and to grow. Mindfulness works best when we choose to take our own lives seriously and to also value the lives of others.

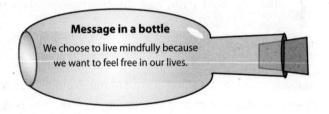

Message in a bottle
We choose to live mindfully because we want to feel free in our lives.

Postscript: beyond depression

This book has tried to reach you in the midst of your confusion and pain, and direct you towards a path to recovery. It has never tried to minimise your pain or make recovery sound like something simple. By offering an understanding of depression, some practical steps to overcome it, and an introduction to the practice of mindfulness as a means to support your recovery and continuing growth, it hopefully has spoken to wherever you find yourself in your life journey.

Recovery does not mean the absence of feeling vulnerable. It means discovering a new strength in yourself that enables you to accept your insecurities, listen to them and learn from them. Someone who has truly recovered from depression is someone who carries within them a greater awareness of how vulnerable they are, but also how this vulnerability can open their hearts and awaken their compassion.

Maturity and inner strength do not mean being on top of things all the time, or feeling good all the time. Strength is about being able to accept how you are feeling at any point in time, including all those times you feel down, and dealing with it in a way that is accepting, compassionate and encouraging. Recovery is about becoming more open with yourself, more spontaneous, and accepting all the different aspects of your personality. The key is learning to live gently with yourself and to be attentive to the things that matter most to you in your life.

Revisiting and rewriting this book has given me the

opportunity to share some insights that have become clearer to me since the first edition was published over 10 years ago. In that time, there has been something of an evolution in our collective appreciation about the importance of mental health generally. People are becoming less afraid to talk about the challenges they experience in their emotional and interpersonal lives. There is a greater awareness of how vulnerable we all are to becoming depressed and many programmes and therapies have been developed to give people the skills to navigate their way through periods of crisis in their lives.

Sometimes, there is a tendency in current self-help literature to regard depression as something 'wrong' that we must 'fix' at all costs. What I have tried to communicate in this book is that depression does not reflect something broken in us, but rather the need within us to grow through facing the stresses and vulnerabilities in our lives. When it becomes intense, we may well need to draw on a range of professional expertise to support us and to get us back on our feet. But, ultimately, we come to terms with, and recover from, depression when we are willing to learn from the experience, rather than view it as an enemy that we have to expel from our lives.

To conclude, I would like to quote for the last time from Sarah's journal. After a difficult struggle with depression, she recovered a strong sense of herself and felt happier in herself than she had ever remembered. Like many people, Sarah's honesty with herself and her courage to persist through the confusion of depression were an inspiration to all who had the privilege of assisting her in her journey.

Sarah's recovery journal

Conclusion

Recovery takes time. It takes all the time you've got. It starts when you realise that you are depressed and you are willing to change how you feel. And it's that will that keeps you going. It vanishes every so often, but reappears so gently at times and so strong at others because you really want to be you. You want to be the hidden you, who secretly you know is wonderful, but who you're afraid to be in case it doesn't work out. But taking those risks and allowing yourself time gets you there. It's not easy to fight with the thoughts that keep you chained to depression. It's a long and difficult struggle, but it's worthwhile.

Depression is not something that 'got me', or 'trapped me' or 'smothered me'. I wasn't at the mercy of depression, I was at the mercy of myself and the young innocent girl within me, who had tried her best all of her life but who felt that she could never get it right. I have spent time with that young girl, and I have spent time in therapy, and I take medication, and I write in a journal and I now spend time with the people in my world whom I want to spend time with. I have a better understanding of myself now, and I like who I am.

I won't ever say I'm glad to have experienced depression, but I wouldn't know what I know now if I hadn't gone through it. I've come a long way from some very dark moments and from painful days of despair. The pain doesn't completely vanish, it eases and it lessens as you start to understand it.

I always had a feeling, that there was something special in me, I always suspected it. And now I'm beginning to see what that special thing is. It's me, it's being me. It's being Sarah as

COMING THROUGH DEPRESSION

she's never been before. It's feeling what I feel and understanding my feelings. Most of all, it's the beginning of caring about me and looking after myself and allowing myself to do so.

And there are times throughout the day when I feel a warmth inside me for what seems like no apparent reason. It's these moments, which are so precious for me, when I feel happy, relaxed and content as I realise just how precious life is. I'm glad to be alive!

References and resources

Barks, C. & Moyne, J. (1997). *The Essential Rumi.* San Francisco, CA: HarperCollins.

Bates, T. & Scanlan, F. (2008). The DEORA Mindfulness Programme: A pilot study to explore the benefits of mindfulness training for people recovering from addiction. Dublin: Headstrong, www.headstrong.ie.

Begikhani, N. (2007). *Bells of Speech.* London: Ambit Books.

Burns, D. D. (1999). *The Feeling Good Handbook.* London: Penguin.

Gilbert, P. (2007). *Overcoming Depression: A Guide to Recovery with a Complete Self-Help Programme.* London: Robinson.

Hanh, T. N. (1975). *The Miracle of Mindfulness.* Boston, MA: Beacon Press.

Hanh, T. N. (2000). *The Path of Emancipation: Talks from a 21-day Mindfulness Retreat.* Berkeley, CA: Parallax Press.

Kabat-Zinn, J. (1990). *Full Catastrophe Living.* New York, NY: Random House.

Kingsolver, B. (1995). *High Tide in Tucson: Essays from Now or Never.* London: HarperCollins.

Miller, W. R. & Seligman, M. E. P. (1975). 'Depression and learned helplessness in man'. *Journal of Abnormal Psychology,* 84, 228–38.

Nye, S. N. (1994). *Words Under the Words: Selected Poems.* Portland, OR: Eighth Mountain Press.

Segal, Z., Teasdale, J. & Williams, M. (2002). *Mindfulness-Based Cognitive Therapy for Depression.* New York, NY: Guilford Press.

Welwood, J. (2002). *Toward a Psychology of Awakening: Buddhism, Psychotherapy, and the Path of Personal and Spiritual Transformation.* Boston, MA and London: Shambhala.

Winnicott, D. W. (1963). 'The Value of Depression'. In: C. Winnicot, R. & Shepherd, M. David (eds), *Home is Where we Start From: Essays of a Psychoanalyst* (1986). London: Penguin Books.

Further reading on depression

Terry Lynch (2004). *Beyond Prozac: Healing Mental Distress* (2nd edition), PCCS: Ross-on-Wye, UK.

This is a very readable and thought-provoking book. Terry Lynch, himself a medical doctor with 18 years' experience, is convinced that doctors prescribe tranquilisers and anti-depressants far too easily. This book sets out to show that while medication has a place, it is only part of the solution. Terry Lynch cites many interesting case histories which show that patients gained far more by having someone who would listen and not judge or blame them, who made them feel safe, and who completely accepted that there are very good reasons why someone might feel depressed or indeed suicidal. This is a very compassionate book and is a must for anyone who has themself or whose family and/or friends have ever struggled with depression or anxiety.

Andrew Solomon (2001). *The Noonday Demon: An Atlas of Depression.* New York, NY: A Touchstone Book.

This book takes the reader on a somewhat academic but fascinating trip across different cultures to explore how human beings have tried to make sense of and treat depression through history. Andrew Solomon weaves what he learns into his own very personal journey to come to terms with very severe episodes of depression. His account of his own experiences are at times harrowing, but they are also tinged with wit and insights that ultimately make this book a hopeful account of the power we have within us to survive our demons.

Gwyneth Lewis (2002). *Sunbathing in the Rain: A cheerful book about depression*. London: Flamingo.

Lewis takes us through the few highs and many lows of a depression that left her dead to the world in her late thirties. She examines the triggers for the depression – alarm bells ringing on the hormonal clock, struggling with two careers as a BBC administrator and poet, and a crisis of confidence in her poetry. She tells us that she is genetically susceptible – her mother's depression threw a silent curse over her childhood.

Lewis shows how she struggled for energy, for breath, for hope when she became depressed. She writes with stark clarity about the darkness, the silence and the misery of depression. About how lost to yourself you can become: 'You are so bereft of personality that even if you wanted to hang yourself you couldn't find a self to hang.' Perhaps not as much cheer here as you might expect from the title, but a very honest and poetic account of the experience nonetheless.

Dorothy Lowe (1996). *Depression: The way out of your prison* (2nd edition). London: Routledge.

An easily understandable and comforting book by therapist and author Dorothy Rowe. The technical content of the book is minimised, so those seeking a biochemical or genetic analysis must go to another source. The author may have feared that some readers would come to view depression as a purely chemical problem, and therefore beyond their control.

Depression described only as a biochemical imbalance would also suggest chemical solutions, which the author personally dislikes.

Melanie Fennell (1999). *Overcoming Low Self-Esteem*. London: Constable & Robinson.

This is an incredibly well-written account of the nature of low self-esteem and the power of destructive thinking patterns that so easily take our minds hostage. It is a very practical book aimed at giving the reader lots of exercises and experiments to restore their sense of personal control and boost their self-esteem. This book is written in a warm, friendly and comforting tone. The author was one of the most talented clinical supervisors I have ever encountered and also one of the more compassionate human beings I have met, particularly with people who struggled with severe depression. She clearly shows us that compassion for oneself (instead of putting yourself down) is essential to your recovery, and she explains we may have developed certain unhelpful thought patterns, and how we can begin to undo them.

Mark Williams, John Teasdale, Zindel Segal & Jon Kabat-Zinn (2007). *The Mindful Way through Depression: Freeing yourself from chronic unhappiness*. New York, NY: Guilford Press.

This superb book brings together the four pioneers of the mindfulness-based training courses and describes clearly the key elements of these courses when applied to helping prevent relapse with people who are vulnerable to depression.

The book is divided into four sections. The first gives a clear account of depression, how it is perpetuated and how mindfulness can help to break the cycle. Part two introduces mindfulness practices, especially those focusing on breathing. There is an emphasis on the acceptance of mental distractions –

or 'mind waves' as they are referred to – as natural and inevitable. Moreover, distractions are presented as ideal learning opportunities; when a person is caught up in something, they can learn how to disengage and so become more familiar with the experience of not being caught up. This section also teaches how mindfulness can offer an alternative to unhelpful rumination, which plays a key part in exacerbating depression. Part three focuses on feelings, emotions and thoughts, and on practising mindfulness in everyday life. The final section of the book brings the different elements together and describes the eight-week course. There is also a CD of meditation exercises guided by Kabat-Zinn.

Paul Gilbert (2007). *Overcoming Depression: A guide to recovery with a complete self-help programme*. London: Constable & Robinson.

This book offers a very original understanding of depression. Paul Gilbert views depression from a biological/evolutionary perspective. As one reader wrote: 'Mr Gilbert offers for depression is something I have encountered nowhere else, yet is so basic and elemental and makes complete sense. This book clarified and simplified what was for me a dark, scary, overwhelming mystery, and helped me to finally see depression for what it is. I understand now that I'm not randomly and unfortunately afflicted with a strange disease that I'm powerless to affect, but rather all people have the potential to enter a depressed state, and similarly all people, including me, have the potential to live in a state of vitality.'

David Burns (1999). *The Feeling Good Handbook*. London: HarperCollins.

Over the past 20 years, cognitive-behavioural therapy has become the predominant form of therapy practised by psychologists.

Burns is one of the biggest popularisers of CBT.

Burns takes a very simple approach – he does not place any weight on diagnostic categories or figuring out 'why' people behave the way they do or the roots of their problems, instead, every depressed thought is traced to irrational thought processes. Why those thought processes were developed is less important to him than being able to recognise self-defeating thought patterns and challenge them. In many ways, I feel this book simplifies the challenge of resolving depression, but I also have to say that is one of its key strengths. It is written in a clear, readable and highly engaging manner and communicates great confidence to the reader, that they have what it takes to recover.

Mark Williams and Danny Penman (2011). *Mindfulness: A Practical Guide to Finding Peace in a Frantic World*. London: Piatkus Books.

Mindfulness reveals a set of simple yet powerful practices that you can weave into your daily life to help break the cycle of unhappiness, stress, anxiety and mental exhaustion. The book is based on Mindfulness-Based Cognitive Therapy (MBCT), which has been clinically proven to be at least as effective as drugs for depression and is recommended by the UK's National Institute of Clinical Excellence. More importantly, it also works for people who are not depressed but who are struggling to keep up with the constant demands of the modern world. Mindfulness focuses on promoting joy and peace rather than banishing unhappiness. It is precisely focused to help ordinary people boost their happiness and confidence levels whilst also reducing anxiety, stress and irritability.

Further reading on mindfulness

Chodron, P. (2000). *When Things Fall Apart: Heart Advice for Difficult Times*. Boston, MA and London: Shambhala.

Crane, R. (2009). *Mindfulness-Based Cognitive Therapy.* London: Routledge.

Epstein, M. (1995). *Thoughts without a Thinker: Psychotherapy from a Buddhist Perspective.* New York, NY: Basic Books.

Germen, C. K., Siegel, R. D. & Fulton, P. R. (2005). *Mindfulness and Psychotherapy.* New York, NY: Guilford Press.

Gunaratana, B. (2002). *Mindfulness in Plain English.* Somerville, MA: Wisdom Publications.

Hayes, S. C., Strosahl, K. D. & Wilson, K. G. (1999). *Acceptance and Commitment Therapy: An Experiential Approach to Behavior Change.* New York, NY: Guilford Press.

Hayes, S. C., Follette, V. M. & Linehan, M. M. (eds) (2004). *Mindfulness and Acceptance: Expanding the Cognitive-Behavioral Tradition.* New York, NY: Guilford Press.

Kabat-Zinn, J. (1994). *Wherever You Go There You Are: Mindfulness Meditation in Everyday Life.* New York, NY: Hyperion.

Kabat-Zinn, J. (2005). *Coming to Our Senses: Healing Ourselves and the World through Mindfulness.* New York, NY: Hyperion.

Kennedy, Sister Stan (2006). *Stillness.* Dublin: TownHouse & CountryHouse.

Kornfield, J. (1993). *A Path with Heart: A Guide through the Perils and Promises of Spiritual Life.* New York, NY: Bantam.

Mace, C. (2008). *Mindfulness and Mental Health.* London: Routledge.

Magio, B. (2008). *Ending the Pursuit of Happiness: A Zen Guide.* Boston, MA: Wisdom Publications.

Martin, P. (2000). *The Zen Path through Depression.* San Francisco, CA: HarperCollins.

Merton, T. (2004). *The Inner Experience: Notes on Contemplation.* San Francisco, CA: HarperCollins.

Rinpoche, S. (2002). *The Tibetan Book of Living and Dying.* London: Rider & Co.

Williams, M. and Penman, D. (2011). *Mindfulness: A Practical Guide to Finding Peace in a Frantic World.* London: Piatkus Books.

Williams, M., Teasdale, J., Segal, Z. & Kabat-Zinn, J. (2007). *The Mindful Way through Depression: Freeing yourself from Chronic Unhappiness.* New York, NY: Guilford Press.

Websites

Courses and meetings in Ireland:
www.mindfulness-ireland.org/

Mindfulness-based stress reduction:
www.umassmed.edu/cfm

Dialectal behaviour therapy:
www.behavioraltech.com
Acceptance and commitment therapy:
www.acceptanceandcommitmenttherapy.com

Institute for Meditation and Psychotherapy:
www.meditationandpsychotherapy.org

Audiovisual materials of all kinds:
www.soundstrue.com

Mindfulness teacher talks:
www.dharmaseed.org

Journal for mindfulness practitioners:
www.inquiringmind.com

Thich Nhat Hanh link:
www.iamhome.org

Resources and support organisations

AWARE – www.aware.ie

The website of Aware, a national voluntary organisation that aims to support people who are experiencing depression, contains information and tips on coping with depression. It also contains details of support groups and services for people with depression.

BODYWHYS – www.bodywhys.ie

The website of the national voluntary organisation Bodywhys aims to support individuals and their families in relation to eating disorders. The site has information and links to services and supports, including details of a lo-call helpline.

GROW – www.grow.ie

GROW is a voluntary mental-health organisation that aims to support people who have suffered, or are suffering, from mental health problems. Details of the organisation are available on its website.

HEADSTRONG – www.headstrong.ie

This is a national organisation committed to changing how Ireland thinks about young people and their mental health, and to establishing youth-friendly accessible supports for all young people in their local communities, called Jigsaw. Specific information regarding Jigsaw services can be accessed via www.jigsaw.ie.

HEADSPACE TOOLKIT WEBSITE – www.headspaceireland.ie

A Mental Health Commission website with information and downloads for young people who are inpatients in mental-health facilities that is aimed at ensuring young people are included in the decisions that affect them and that their rights are upheld.

Downloads include resource packs with information for young people to use.

LET SOMEONE KNOW – www.letsomeoneknow.ie

A Health Service Executive website aimed at promoting mental health and help-seeking in young people. It includes tips for young people on how to look after their mental health.

MENTAL HEALTH IRELAND – www.mentalhealthireland.ie

Mental Health Ireland is a national voluntary organisation with 104 local Mental Health Associations (MHAs) and branches throughout the country. MHI aims to promote positive mental health and to actively support persons with mental-health difficulties, their families and carers by identifying their needs and advocating their rights.

OCD IRELAND – www.ocdireland.org

OCD Ireland's website has information and links for people with obsessive compulsive disorder and other related difficulties.

PIETA HOUSE: CENTRE FOR THE PREVENTION OF SUICIDE OR SELF-HARM – www.pieta.ie

Pieta House offers a support and counselling service for people who self-harm or feel suicidal.

REACHOUT.COM – www.reachout.com

This website is an online mental-health resource that provides high-quality mental-health fact sheets and a detailed overview of the range of informal and formal mental-health supports available in Ireland. ReachOut.com also engages young people by publishing personal stories about getting through tough times and finding the support and inspiration to face up to and overcome mental health difficulties.

SAMARITANS – www.samaritans.org

The Samaritans is an organisation that provides confidential, non-judgemental, emotional support, 24 hours a day for people who are experiencing feelings of distress or despair, including those which could lead to suicide.

SHINE – www.shine.ie

Shine is a national, voluntary organisation that supports people and their families who are experiencing long-term mental-health difficulties. There is information on the site about the support services offered by Shine as well as an information helpline number.

YOUR MENTAL HEALTH – www.yourmentalhealth.ie

A Health Service Executive website that provides information on looking after your mental health.

1LIFE – www.1life.ie

1Life provides a 24-hour suicide prevention and intervention helpline providing professional counselling services for anyone who has an issue related to suicide, whether an individual in suicidal crisis or a person seeking advice or information on behalf of another. 1Life provides a freephone telephone counselling service as well as text and cyber counselling.

Permission acknowledgments

'Calm' by Nazand Begikhani reprinted by kind permission of the author.

'Kindness' from *Words Under Words* by Naomi Shihab Nye courtesy of The Eighth Mountain Press.

'The Guest House' by Rumi, translated by Coleman Barks, reprinted by kind permission of the translator.

Index